THE FITNESS FACTOR

Every Woman's Key to a Lifetime of Health and Well-Being

THE FITNESS FACTOR

Every Woman's Key to a Lifetime of Health and Well-Being

Lisa Callahan, M.D.

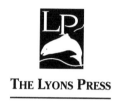

THE LYONS PRESS

Guilford, Connecticut
An imprint of The Globe Pequot Press

The Lyons Press is an imprint of The Globe Pequot Press.

Printed in the United States of America

10 9 8 7 6 5 4 3 2 1

Design by Compset, Inc.

Library of Congress Cataloging-in-Publication Data

Callahan, Lisa.
    The fitness factor : every woman's key to a lifetime of health and well-being / Lisa Callahan.
        p. cm.
    Includes index.
    ISBN 1-58574-501-4
        1. Exercise for women. 2. Physical fitness for women. 3. Women—Health and hygiene.
    I. Title.

RA778 .C2146 2002
613.7'045—dc21
                                                                    2001050729

In memory of September 11, 2001

ACKNOWLEDGMENTS

THIS BOOK IS the fulfillment of a personal dream, one that could not have come true without the support of many people. I am deeply grateful to my colleagues and the staff of the Women's Sports Medicine Center, especially Jo Hannafin, M.D., Ph.D.; Deborah Saint-Phard, M.D.; Pamela Sherman, M.D.; and Robyn Stuhr, M.A. Special recognition must go to Robyn, who painstakingly reviewed the entire manuscript and provided invaluable insights and suggestions, as well as constant and enthusiastic encouragement. Nellie Alfalla and Miriam Blanco kept my office running smoothly while I was immersed in writing. I owe many thanks to the administration of the Hospital for Special Surgery, especially Russell F. Warren, M.D.

While there is not enough space on this page to thank my many mentors, three deserve special mention: Jeff Tanji, M.D.,

Martin Trieb, M.D., and Jim Colville, M.D. These men taught me much of what I know about sports medicine, never inhibited by the fact that at the time they took me under their collective wings, I was a woman in what was generally still considered to be a man's world. I am also enormously indebted to those who continue to teach me on a daily basis, my patients.

Thanks to Becky Koh, my patient and thoughtful editor, and Kris Dahl, my terrific agent, for believing in this book from its conception. And last but not least, I'd like to thank my family, especially my father, to whom I owe my love of exercise and the great outdoors, and my mother, from whom I learned that all things are possible. My deepest gratitude is to Mark, my wonderful husband and fitness partner; without his constant love and support, this book might still be just a dream.

CONTENTS

Contents

Contents

Contents

INTRODUCTION

As THE COFOUNDER and medical director of the country's first women's sports medicine center, I am frequently asked why there is a need for a facility dedicated to promoting medical care, research, and education of athletic women. I find it fascinating that of the many times I've heard this question, it has never been asked by an active woman. The active woman knows all too well the reasons.

Like many sports medicine physicians, I came to my interest in sports medicine naturally: as an avid recreational athlete who has seen her share of injuries. Most of the time, I simply walked them off, waited them out, or continued to exercise while injured. On occasion, an injury forced me to see a physician, like the time I tore a ligament in my knee while skating, fractured a rib playing hockey, and badly strained a hamstring while running. I was given X rays and pain pills, but no advice. No one ever talked to me about training correctly, choosing the right equipment, or rehabilitating my injuries. I knew nothing about the impact of nutrients like iron, calcium, and carbohydrates on my athletic performance, or on my overall health. I had nowhere and no one to turn to with questions about exercise and my menstrual cycle, weight training and building muscle, or why I chronically had heel blisters from my running shoes. When I looked for answers, I simply found more questions.

As frustrating as these experiences were, they also provided me with the inspiration that would shape my professional future. During my own search for information, I found other active women looking for answers to questions I had not yet even considered. Could exercise help prevent breast cancer? Is weight lifting safe during pregnancy? Why are certain injuries more common in women than in men? Could exercise delay the usual effects of aging?

After completing training in family medicine and sports medicine, I began to focus my medical practice on active women. I took care of female athletes from local high schools and two universities, as well as recreational athletes of all ages. In 1994, I had the good fortune of meeting Dr. Jo Hannafin, an orthopedic surgeon and world-class rower. Together, we created the Women's Sports Medicine Center at the Hospital for Special Surgery in New York City. My patients—women of all ages, fitness levels, and backgrounds—have shared with me their victories, goals, concerns, and misconceptions regarding physical fitness and sports. I have watched them exercise through pregnancy, after heart attacks, and during cancer therapy. I've seen them lose weight, lower their blood pressure, and drop cholesterol levels through exercise. I've noticed improvements in osteoporosis and depression because of exercise. I've watched, listened, and learned a great deal. And I have come to believe that *exercise is the single most important choice a woman can make to maximize her health.*

SPREADING THE MESSAGE

When I speak to groups of women about the tremendous impact exercise has on health, at least one skeptical woman usually asks, "If exercise is all that important, why hasn't my doctor made a bigger deal out of it?" The answer may lie in medical history.

If We Knew Then What We Know Now

Knowing what we do in the twenty-first century about the many health benefits of exercise, it's ironic to realize that historically, many of the earlier barriers against women's participation in athletics were erected by doctors. Records from ancient civilizations show that women actively engaged in competitive sports. However, medical writings from the late 1800s portrayed women as fragile, prone to injury and illness. Doctors believed that physical activity could compromise a woman's health and fertility. During the Victorian era, essentially all illnesses in women, from headaches to heart disease, were viewed in relationship to the reproductive organs. Everything was either blamed on a woman's reproductive system or seen as posing a threat to it. Women were treated as invalids during their pregnancies and menstrual cycles. It was believed that any exertion, physical or mental, could harm the uterus.

This type of thinking by doctors and others created the Victorian view of women as inherently fragile, delicate creatures who easily became ill and indisposed. Of course, now that we understand how important physical activity is for optimal health, it is easy to see that the inactive lifestyles of these women would have helped to create a self-fulfilling prophecy. Their lack of physical fitness would have made even simple activities seem strenuous, reinforcing the concept that they were weak. It also would have made for more difficult pregnancies, labor, and childbirth, and would leave them more vulnerable to illness.

The Beginning of Change

It all began to change for women at the turn of the twentieth century, due, at least in part, to two completely unrelated factors: war and the introduction of the bicycle. During World War I, when men headed off to Europe to fight, women took their places working in factories. They began to create sports teams with their fellow female coworkers. During World War II, even more women entered the workforce, often performing jobs requiring significant physical strength. When the wars were over, women were encouraged to return home, leaving those jobs to men. But two significant changes had occurred: women had shattered the myth that they were incapable of performing physically demanding jobs, and they refused to give up their more physically active lifestyles. Because of the popularity of bicycling, they even had their first "sports clothes"—bloomers—which allowed them finally to break free of the cumbersome petticoats, corsets, and starched skirts they had previously worn for all activities.

Unfortunately, women who participated in sports competitions had to keep fighting against "medical wisdom." Doctors continued to assert that participating in competitive sports would have dire health and reproductive consequences. In the 1920s, after a female runner collapsed at the finish line of the first women's 800-meter Olympic race, doctors gravely warned about women's lack of capabilities for performing such "strenuous" events (800 meters is a half mile). They pointed to women's smaller hearts and lungs, saying that women were not capable of meeting the physical demands of the race. The event was dropped from the Olympics, and for *thirty years* women were not allowed to compete in any races longer than 200 meters (one-eighth of a mile).

There is no doubt that such misguided medical views contributed to women being barred from other sports venues, including participation in endurance events such as the marathon. The belief that women weren't physically capable of running 26.2 miles was supported by many medical experts. It was not until 1967, when pioneer Kathrine Switzer covertly entered and successfully completed the then men's-only Boston Marathon, that women were allowed to enter marathon races. It is astonishing to realize that although men have been competing in the Olympic marathon for hundreds of years, women have had that opportunity only since 1984, less than twenty years!

Where We Are Today

Given this glimpse of history, it should surprise no one that the first Surgeon General's report on physical activity, published just a few years ago, found that more men than women are physically active. Throughout our history, exercise has been actively encouraged in boys and men, but discouraged in girls and women. We have only recently begun to realize how much women's physical capabilities have been misinterpreted and underestimated. Now, of course, we recognize that the Victorian era doctors were wrong. *Not only do women have the physical stamina to exercise and play sports, their health benefits tremendously when they do.*

Because this realization is still so new, we have only uncovered the tip of the iceberg in finding ways that exercise can be used to prevent and treat the diseases—like osteoporosis, diabetes, breast cancer, osteoarthritis, and depression—that are so common in women. Every day, we learn more about how different types of exercise have complementary effects on a woman's body. For instance, some woman are aware that exercise is helpful in reducing the risk of osteoporosis, but they don't know that it is a combination of strength training, weight-bearing aerobic exercise, and balance-training exercises that are most effective. Similarly, many women with arthritis think exercise will just make their joints ache more, and don't know that stretching exercises and low-impact aerobic activity not only relieve pain but preserve joint range of motion.

As proof of the many health benefits of exercise continues to mount, so do women's interest and curiosity. Many want to take more responsibility for their own health and understand they can do this by becoming more physically fit, but don't know where to begin. Others have gotten stuck in exercise "ruts" and don't know how to add to their fitness programs to attain maximal health benefits. Still others have fallen into the trap of "more is better" and don't understand the negative health consequences of overexercise. The abundance of fitness myths and misinformation women have been exposed to, coupled with society's emphasis on exercise for weight loss, is mind-boggling!

This book grew out of my professional experiences, as well as my personal ones. It is my hope that it will answer a few questions, dispel a few myths, and point every woman in the direction of better health through fitness. I believe that we've entered an exciting era in the medical world, wherein the best medicine a doctor may recommend to you is not a new pill, but a pair of walking shoes, a yoga class, or a weight bench. But don't wait! Whether you have already been diagnosed with an illness or want to try to prevent one, the time to start a smart exercise program is *right now*. You can develop your own fitness prescription, one that will be a powerful insurance plan for a lifetime of wellness. This book will show you how.

PART 1

WHAT'S YOUR EXERCISE ATTITUDE?

CHAPTER 1

THE EXERCISE CHALLENGE

Imagine picking up the morning paper and seeing the front-page banner headline:

Miraculous New Anti-Aging Pill Discovered

You scan the article, which reports that this new miracle drug can increase your energy, make you look younger, decrease your risk of serious illness such as heart disease and breast cancer, all with no side effects! You'd probably rush right out to stand in line at your local drugstore for a lifetime supply of this amazing new medication. Of course, this pill has not yet been discovered, and despite the miracles of modern medicine, I can assure you that it's not likely to arrive any time soon. However, there is something already available to every one of us that can provide all of these benefits and more. It's exercise.

WHY EXERCISE IS THE BEST MEDICINE FOR A LIFETIME OF WELLNESS

It's been my experience that a great number of women understand the goal of exercise to be purely cosmetic improvement. They view the benefits of exercise as equal to the benefits of, say, plastic surgery—as a tool we use to change the way we look. And why shouldn't they think this? Pick up any women's magazine, and the headline tells the story: "Go Sleeveless! Sexy Arms in Just 4 Weeks"; "Exercise Emergency: The Bikini Workout"; "Love Your Legs: Uncover Long, Lean, Sexy Muscles"; "The Secret to Perfect Abs/Butt/Thighs"; "Shortcuts to the Sexy Body You Deserve."

I've yet to meet a woman who wouldn't like to have the fantasy body promised by such articles, but most of them are too busy with real life to do more than scan the headlines. It's no wonder that exercise drops to the bottom of a woman's to-do list, right above "get a manicure" and "take a bubble bath." *We need to change the way we think about exercise.* The truth is that women who exercise:

lower their risk of cancer
are less likely to suffer a heart attack
sleep better
have increased energy
experience less depression
report better sex lives
decrease their risk of osteoporosis
have healthier pregnancies
have clearer, smoother skin
drop their cholesterol levels
spend less money on health care
have better posture
are less likely to smoke

improve their mental alertness and concentration
report lower levels of stress
slash their risk of developing diabetes
are less likely ever to need prescription medications

You can get these health benefits from exercise no matter what your age, but surprisingly, women in their thirties and older stand to reap some of exercise's greatest rewards. This is because the human body's functions need a boost after thirty or so years of use. Even the most sophisticated machines eventually start to show signs of wear and tear, and the human body is no different. And while many women turn to the expensive (and sometimes risky) option of plastic surgery to retain a youthful appearance, such a solution is only skin deep. Plastic surgery may make us look younger, but it can't do a thing to make us feel younger or live healthier for longer. Exercise, however, can age-proof us from the inside out.

ARE YOU TOO BUSY FOR YOUR OWN GOOD?

Despite all of the known health benefits of exercise, only 15 percent to 20 percent of adult women exercise on a regular basis many of them do so for cosmetic reasons. Why don't more women take advantage of the health benefits of exercise?

Believe it or not, the most common theme among the thousands of women I've talked to is that "exercise costs too much." Often this perceived cost is not measured in dollars, but rather in *time*. Women today are busier than ever. While most of my patients understand in a kind of abstract way that they "should" exercise, they spend so much time taking care of everyone and everything else—families, homes, jobs—that exercise gets shoved aside as an optional activity or, worse, an unaffordable luxury.

The second most common reason women say they don't exercise is that they're too exhausted by their other commitments. As one harried patient put it, "I'm too tired to even *think* about exercising!" Other popular excuses include:

"There's no one to watch the kids."
"I don't like to sweat."
"I can't afford a gym."
"I'll make a fool of myself."

While I'm sympathetic to the enormous number of daily demands each of us faces, it essentially boils down to one simple fact: *Women can't afford NOT to exercise.*

LOOKING FOR A BARGAIN? THE PRICE OF EXERCISE IS RIGHT

If you're one of the many women who say, "I don't have time or energy to exercise," you don't understand what a terrific bargain you're passing up. Isn't preventing a heart attack worth a few hours of your time? What is decreasing your risk of developing cancer worth to you? How much would you give to be in good enough health to dance at your grandchild's wedding?

If good health came with a guarantee, I'm betting most of us would pay any price asked. Obviously that will never happen, but you can take out an insurance policy of sorts in the form of exercise. Since exercise is one of the most effective ways you can safeguard your health from a tremendous number of diseases, it's really an investment in a lifetime of wellness. And a little can go a long way: contrary to what you may think, it doesn't take much of an investment to begin collecting the benefits of exercise. When I work with patients who don't exercise at all, I ask them to commit just *one or two hours a week* for four weeks to beginning an exercise program. They are often amazed at how little it takes to begin reaping the initial benefits of exercise, like improved energy, stress relief, and better sleep. As they continue exercising, they not only begin to see a variety of additional health benefits, they consistently report that exercise makes them feel good as well as look good, and gives them a new sense of empowerment in many aspects of their lives. Viewed that way, a few hours a week spent exercising seems like a real bargain!

And last but not least: Finding the time and energy to exercise is also a question of priorities. Almost every woman I know tends to prioritize the needs of others above her own. I'm willing to bet that whenever there's something extra to be done (Who's going to pick up the kids after soccer practice? Who's going to stay and finish the company report? Who's going to go with Grandma to her doctor's appointment?), you probably take a look at your overbooked life and, lo and behold, manage to find the time to accomplish that important task.

So, here's the challenge: Stop thinking of exercise as a luxury, something that can be bumped to the bottom of the to-do list. Instead, remind yourself that it's a *necessity* that needs to be a priority in your life. Think of it this way: The healthier, more rested, less stressed, and more energetic you become through physical fitness, the better able you'll be to care for all of those various responsibilities in your life. It's like money in the bank.

TODAY, A PUSH-UP . . . TOMORROW, THE WORLD

Mary, a widow in her sixties, came to see me with complaints of fatigue and weakness. Medically, she was healthy, but years of inactivity had resulted in a profound loss of physical fitness. So when she made simple demands of her body, such as carrying two bags of groceries at once, she simply didn't have the muscle strength to do it. Imagine not being able to carry two bags of groceries! Mary was on her way to losing her independence.

Because women, on average, live almost seven years longer than men, many find themselves in Mary's situation—alone, and increasingly unable to care for themselves. Often these women end up in nursing homes—a thought abhorrent to most of us. One recently published report found that 80 percent of women surveyed said they would "rather be dead" than in a nursing home.

Mary was astounded to learn that her failing health was simply the result of a sedentary lifestyle. The thought of losing her independence was a wake-up call, and Mary decided she would do whatever she could to maintain her independent way of life. She committed to an exercise program and was hardly recognizable when she came into the office a few months later. It wasn't just the changes in her physical appearance—such as her improved posture, brisker walk, and leaner body—that were striking, but the changes that had taken place within. She told me that the day she completed a set of push-ups for the first time she cried tears of joy and amazement over her newfound strength.

In just a few short months the fatigue and weakness she initially came to see me about had disappeared. Mary's new exercise program decreased her risk of many of the diseases associated with inactivity, like heart disease, osteoporosis, and high blood pressure. But, equally important, exercise helped to alleviate the depression she had suffered since her husband's death. Taking control of her physical health had encouraged her to take control of her mental and emotional health as well. It gave her the courage to join a support group for women who had lost their husbands, which may be one of the most important things she could have done to improve her health. Studies show that women involved in support groups (including those for weight loss, dealing with cancer or infertility, and substance abuse) often have better success in achieving their goals. To this day, Mary credits exercise with changing her life.

IT'S ABOUT WINNING, NOT LOSING

JOANNE, A FORTY-YEAR-OLD MOTHER of three, wanted to lose the extra fifty pounds she had gained during her pregnancies. She wasn't sure what to do, but she had gotten plenty of advice. Her sources of information—television talk shows, magazine articles, books, celebrities, friends, and relatives—had suggested she eat more protein, eat less protein, avoid carbohydrates, lift weights, not lift weights, exercise daily, exercise twice daily, and fast without exercising at all. She tried several diets but only ended up gaining back the pounds she lost—plus a few more. Her favorite movie stars all seemed to have elaborate exercise programs designed by personal trainers. Her sister recommended aerobics classes, but her best friend thought yoga would be better. Her doctor said, "Try walking."

Joanne couldn't decide what to do. Feeling overwhelmed and increasingly uncertain, she ended up not doing anything at all. By the time she came to see me for advice, her doctor had informed her that her weight had caused her blood pressure to skyrocket, increasing her risk of stroke or heart attack.

THE "WIN-WIN" SOLUTION

When Joanne came to see me, she rattled off the names of several popular diet and exercise programs and then asked which of them was "the best." She was surprised when I answered "none of them." The problem, I explained, was that none of those plans took her individual needs into account. The best program for Joanne, I told her, was the Joanne Plan: one that reflected her current level of fitness, personal interests, health goals, strengths and weaknesses, and resources. No one-size-fits-all program designed by someone else was ever going to be as effective as one she could create for herself. And, I explained, although it's true that any exercise is better than no exercise, a program designed especially with her in mind meant she could take advantage of our knowledge that *different types of exercise have different health benefits.* All she needed was to clarify her personal goals and learn how to reach them.

Like many women when I ask them about their personal exercise goals, Joanne's initial response was an almost pre-programmed one "I need to lose weight." But as we talked, it became clear that Joanne needed more than an exercise program for weight loss: what she needed was to change her way of *thinking* about both exercise and weight loss. Like many patients, she had always viewed her weight as a cosmetic issue. Although she had long been unhappy with her appearance, she hadn't really considered the health consequences of being overweight until her recent visit to her doctor. Although she now wanted to lower her blood pressure and improve her heart health, she felt anxious and was overwhelmed by the intimidating thought of how much time and effort it would take to lose fifty pounds.

Joanne was making two common mistakes that had to be corrected before she could even get to the starting line of a successful exercise program. First, like a majority of women, she had the all-or-nothing approach to weight loss. While her long-term goal of shedding fifty pounds was important, it would obviously take a long time to reach. Joanne needed to develop attainable short-term goals that would boost her confidence and provide motivation. Instead of focusing on the goal of losing fifty pounds, I suggested Joanne plan to lose just five pounds. Once she had successfully dropped the first five pounds, it would simply be a matter of repeating the process nine more times.

Second, and more important, was Joanne's attitude toward exercise. She viewed it as an unpleasant, time-consuming chore that was a waste of time unless she was guaranteed the desired result of weight loss. Like many women, she didn't realize there was an important connection between exercise and good health *independent of weight loss.* I asked her to forget about the scale for a while and focus instead on the ways she could use exercise to improve her health. Joanne felt enormous relief not to have to focus on the seemingly insurmountable task of weight loss. Concentrating instead on taking responsibility for improving her health actually left her feeling excited about the prospect of exercise. In a matter of minutes she'd changed her primary goal from a "losing" proposition ("I need to lose weight") to a "winning" health strategy ("I want to improve my blood pressure"). She set a short-term goal of exercising for four weeks and then planned to have her blood pressure re-checked. I was able to assure her that if she stuck with an exercise program for her health, some weight loss would naturally follow. For Joanne, that was a "win-win" solution.

WHY DIETS DON'T WORK

When I first met Joanne, she complained that she had tried several diets, only to regain the pounds she'd lost plus a few additional ones. Not surprising, I explained to her, because diets just don't work. Here's why:

Women who don't exercise lose muscle mass *every year*, beginning in their late twenties or early thirties. Muscle is *metabolically active*, meaning that it burns a lot of calories, while fat is *metabolically sluggish*, using hardly any. So any loss of muscle slows the body's metabolism (also known as the metabolic rate). This age-related decline in muscle mass leads to a slow but steady drop in metabolism, and a corresponding increase in weight. Unfortunately in America, the number of us who are overweight or obese is increasing every year. At least half of us are overweight (more women than men), and it's been estimated that at any given time, up to *50 million* Americans and two of every three women are dieting in an effort to shed those excess pounds. We spend upwards of $30 billion every year trying to lose weight.

But dieting without exercise is doomed to fail. Why? Because when you diet to lose weight, you don't just lose fat, you lose precious muscle, too. Let's assume that each pound that you lose through dieting is roughly three-quarters fat and one-quarter muscle. That may not sound too bad until you realize that *losing any muscle automatically decreases your body's ability to burn calories.* For example: if a woman loses twenty pounds through dieting, she loses approximately fifteen pounds of fat and five pounds of muscle. If she wants to maintain that weight loss, she'll have to eat even less, because the loss of five pounds of calorie-burning muscle lowers her metabolic rate. Now she burns 150 to 200 fewer calories every day! *This is the reason most women who diet end up gaining the lost weight back—plus a few pounds more.* And here's the worst part: When the weight is regained, it doesn't come back as fifteen pounds of fat and five pounds of muscle, it comes back as twenty pounds of fat. Now, the poor dieter is back to her initial weight, with less muscle and more fat, and a slower metabolic rate. If she consumes the same amount of food she was eating before she started her diet, she will continue to gain weight. *She'd have been better off if she never started the diet in the first place.* But if she had exercised while she dieted, she could have lost weight while maintaining muscle, boosting her calorie-burning capability, maintaining her metabolism, and improving her health.

DESIGNING YOUR OWN WINNING SOLUTION

Maybe you identify with Joanne, but there's still a negative little voice in your head whining that exercise won't work for you, or that it can't really be that important for you, or that it just won't fit into your schedule. Or maybe it is whispering that you can begin an exercise program "after" (after the next holiday, after your children are older, after you finish a project, etc.). If that's the message from your inner voice, then shush it for just five minutes to focus on yourself in the following way:

1. Stand back and pretend that you are an observer, watching yourself go through your day. What do you see? Someone who feels tired all the time? Is dissatisfied with her appearance? Always feels stressed? Constantly puts pleasure aside to complete chores, and feels anxious about getting it all done?

2. Now think back. Was there a time in your life that you felt more in control? More energetic, healthier, or stronger? Do you remember what it was like to be an active child, reveling in the joy of movement? Would you like to recapture that sense of well-being, of vitality?

3. Now think ahead. Fast-forward to a mental picture of yourself in ten years. What do you see? If you see a happy, fulfilled woman in control of her own health and life, then I'd bet that regular physical activity has been an important part of your life. If that's not the mental picture you see, don't despair! Like the character Mr. Scrooge in Dickens's *A Christmas Carol*, you have the opportunity to make some changes today that will make for a better future. The following three simple steps will get you started on your way to a winning game plan for a fitter, healthier you.

Step One: Take a Good Look in the Mirror

Stand in front of a mirror and take a good look at yourself—but not in the way that you normally would. Instead, learn to look at your body the way that a doctor like me would see you. As a physician, I have developed enormous respect and admiration for the human body, an amazing, complex "machine" that most of us take for granted. As you go through your day, thousands of elaborate processes are occurring throughout your body. The immune system is quietly fighting off cancer-causing cell damage; the kidneys and liver are sorting through billions of molecules, flushing potentially dangerous ones out of your system; cells that function like microscopic repairmen scurry about, fixing injuries to skin, bone, and other tissues. Because the human body functions so efficiently, you don't have to spend any conscious energy on making sure all goes according to schedule . . . which leaves your brain plenty of leisure time to criticize the very body that does all these wonderful things for you. However, although the human body is very powerful, it's not superhuman. It needs your help to continue functioning at its highest possible level.

With that perspective of your body in mind, turn to your mirror and see if you can determine what I would see. Simple observations about posture, eye contact, facial expression, skin appearance, and general muscle tone tell me a great deal about a woman's overall health. Try to view your own body not from a *cosmetic* viewpoint ("my thighs are too big"), but from a *functional* one. Visualize your body performing a task you do daily, such as lifting a bag of groceries, bending down to pick up a child, or climbing the stairs. Now visualize not only what you'd *like to see* but also how you'd *like to feel.* Imagine feeling stronger and completing the task with more energy. See yourself standing taller, skin glowing, body fit and firm. Begin to develop a mental picture of the fit, healthy woman you would like to be.

Step Two: Define Your Health Goals

With the image of yourself as a fit and healthy woman in mind, the next step is to write down all of the improvements in your health that you personally would like to achieve through fitness. One way to get started is to first make a list of diseases and health problems that are prevalent in your family. Does cancer or heart disease or osteoporosis run in your family? Did your grandparents suffer from arthritis? Do you have siblings, aunts, or uncles with diabetes or high blood pressure? We know that most medical conditions result from a combination of factors, including heredity and lifestyle. And although you can't change your genes, you can make lifestyle choices to minimize your risk of developing many diseases and to maximize your health. Use the following list for ideas, but add your own specific goals.

My Health Goals (sample list)

Lower cholesterol
Combat smoking-related damage
Control blood pressure
Prevent diabetes
Manage depression
Avoid a heart attack
Improve bone density
Reduce stress
Have a healthy pregnancy

Step Three: Determine Your Exercise History

Now that you've identified your health and fitness goals, you can best achieve them by understanding how and why exercise went wrong for you in the past. Time and time again I've seen a woman begin a well-intentioned exercise program only to quit soon after, which leaves her feeling that she's "failed" at exercise. In reality, it's usually that the program she chose failed *her,* simply because it was a poor fit for her personally.

(I tell my patients that it's absolutely fine to "try on" the latest celebrity-endorsed workout, but not to be surprised if it doesn't fit their lives any better than the celebrity's clothes would fit their bodies.) Carefully think through the following questions about your personal exercise history, and be honest with yourself when it comes to the answers. This information will lay the foundation for your personalized game plan and will speed you on your way to becoming the woman in your mental picture—the best, healthiest, strongest you can be.

Personal Exercise History Questionnaire

1. In the past 3 years, on average, I have exercised _____ .
   a. 3 times a week or more
   b. 1 to 2 times a week
   c. only occasionally
   d. rarely or never

2. The main reason I haven't exercised more is: (choose as many as apply)
   a. I don't like exercise
   b. I don't have time for exercise
   c. It costs too much money
   d. It's not important to me
   e. I don't have the energy to exercise
   f. Other:

3. Reason(s) I would consider beginning an exercise program include: (choose as many as apply)
   a. to lose weight
   b. to meet new people
   c. to have fun
   d. to spend time with a family member or friend who exercises
   e. to reduce stress
   f. to improve my health
   g. Other:

4. On a separate sheet of paper, list each type of exercise you've tried in the past. Write down what you did or didn't like about each one.

5. Think about how you felt when you were doing an activity you enjoyed. What did you like about it? Why did you stop doing that particular activity? What would allow you to resume that activity, or one similar to it?

6. Close your eyes and imagine a fit, energetic, happy, healthy woman doing a particular activity. Imagine yourself in her place. Now open your eyes. What activity did you just visualize yourself doing?

Interpreting Your Answers

If you answered "a" to question 1, congratulations! You should already be enjoying many of the health benefits of fitness if you perform regular, vigorous exercise at least three times a week. But if exercise has not been a regular part of your routine, don't despair: the less fit you currently are, the faster you will see changes when exercise becomes a consistent part of your life!

The second question is designed to get you thinking about some of the potential barriers to your personal exercise program. *This is an extremely important part of planning your program.* Many women start with good intentions but let daily challenges overcome their commitment to exercise. Over the next few days, think about your answers to this question and begin to imagine yourself enjoying exercise and its benefits. If that nagging voice continues to argue that you can't incorporate exercise into your day, listen to it ... but only long enough to write down its arguments under the heading "Potential Barriers to Reaching My Health Goals." Then silence that voice by developing your own strategies to deal with these possible obstacles. Use the examples in the Overcoming the Obstacles to Exercise section that follows to get started. Be creative! If you can't think of a solution to an identified barrier, ask for help from someone who supports your efforts to get healthier.

Although we have been focusing on the health benefits of exercise, the third question in the personal exercise history questionnaire reminds you of some of the additional advantages of exercise. Think creatively about the possible social benefits of exercise. Maybe you have a friend or neighbor whom you would enjoy seeing more frequently; she could become an exercise buddy. Or maybe your husband has hinted that he'd like it if you joined his coed softball team. Possibly you feel isolated and would enjoy finding an activity that would provide new sources of friendship.

And those social benefits actually have an impact on your health! Studies have shown that women who feel connected to others live longer and get sick less frequently. Other research has shown us that women who exercise together have better success sticking with an exercise plan.

Your answers to the third question as well as to the three that follow it will help you to design your personal exercise program around activities that you'll really enjoy. The side benefit of all that fun? Extra motivation for staying committed to your personal fitness program.

OVERCOMING THE OBSTACLES TO EXERCISE

Women name a tremendous number of obstacles to regular exercise, but with a little creative thinking and planning, they can all be overcome. Some of my most frequent discussions with patients revolve around the following:

Lack of time: This is probably the number one obstacle to regular exercise reported by busy women. Everyone's day has exactly twenty-four hours in it; what is variable is how we *choose* to use those hours. If you can't find time for exercise, you need to reorganize your priorities, putting your personal health right up at the top of the list. Since exercise is one of the most effective ways to pursue optimal health, it needs to fit into your schedule, just like brushing your teeth or eating your fruits and vegetables. If you don't always have thirty consecutive minutes to exercise, spend ten consecutive minutes three times a day in vigorous activity like taking the stairs, gardening, or walking the dog. Don't fight for a parking space near the front of the mall: park far away and walk quickly to the entrance. Mow the lawn in summer; rake the leaves in the fall. Walk briskly around the house doing your daily chores. See how fast you can fold a load of laundry. Who knows, by doing routine tasks at a brisk pace, you may suddenly find yourself with more time for exercise, after all! Make a contract with yourself; or schedule exercise appointments on your calendar, and treat them as if they were doctor appointments (or some other commitment you wouldn't ignore).

Child care needs: This is a commonly identified barrier to a busy woman's commitment to a regular exercise program. Some solutions to this barrier include: finding a gym with child care facilities; establishing a network of mothers who will take turns swapping baby-sitting duties; exercising at home; exercising when the children are in school, or exercising early in the morning or late in the evening when someone else is available to provide child care. (Many women report that their spouses are willing to trade thirty to forty-five minutes a few times a week for a happier, healthier wife!)

JOGGING STROLLERS

Don't let having an infant or toddler at home keep you from a walking or jogging workout: Invest in an exercise stroller. Also called jogging or running strollers, these are the beast-of-burden cousins of your everyday stroller. The three-wheel design is stable and sturdy, and it won't send your precious cargo flying every time you hit a bump. Look for one that folds (so it fits easily into your car or when taking mass transit) and has a sun canopy, a safety wrist strap, and a brake at your fingertips. There is even a "twin" model—wow, what a workout!

Lack of energy: If this sounds like your obstacle, try exercising early in the morning, at lunchtime, or with a friend who won't let you out of your commitment to fitness. Remind yourself that regular exercise will increase your stamina and leave you with more energy. Have a snack before you exercise, preferably a mix of carbohydrate and protein like fruit with yogurt, cheese and an apple, or half a turkey sandwich (see chapter 9: How to Eat Like an Athlete). However, you may want to avoid having a high sugar treat like a candy bar, because the surge of sugar into your bloodstream from such a snack triggers the release of insulin, which then causes your blood sugar to plummet and leaves you more tired than you were to start with.

Lack of money: This is never an excuse not to exercise. Getting fitter and healthier doesn't have to cost you a cent. Consider checking exercise videotapes out of the library, or renting them from a video store. Begin a walking club in your neighborhood or during your lunch hour at work. Look for reduced-rate memberships to gyms: Many offer discounts for off-peak hours or for family or group memberships. Scan the classifieds in the newspaper for good-quality, little-used exercise equipment. Design your exercise program around inexpensive tools like a jump rope, or exercises such as push-ups and sit-ups that don't require any equipment at all.

WHAT DOES FITNESS LOOK LIKE?

Now that you've identified your goals and the potential obstacles to attaining them, it's time to design your personal fitness plan. When you think of a physically fit woman, whom do you picture? Maybe a gold medal–winning Olympic athlete or an aerobics instructor at the gym or your slender neighbor. Although fitness comes in many shapes and sizes, you may be surprised to find that thin does not equal fit, and that there is not a real consensus on exactly how to measure physical fitness. For such a simple little word, the concept of *fitness* still provokes a lot of discussion. Are you fit if you can run a mile in ten minutes? Hold a yoga pose? Lift a heavy weight? Stay the same weight you were in college? Some health experts see fitness as a "quality of life" issue. In other words, being fit means being active and healthy, and getting the most out of life. There's plenty of room for you to decide what fitness means to you.

As a physician, I think of fitness as the sum of four components that, together, allow the human body to function at its best. These four components are *cardiovascular capacity, muscular strength and endurance, flexibility,* and *body composition.* In simple English, this means that your heart is powerful and healthy; your muscles are strong and capable; your joints have normal motion; and your body has a healthy amount of fat—not too much, not too little. It's important to understand how each of these aspects of fitness contributes to better health. Although you can improve your well-being by focusing on any one of these components of fitness, the best way to boost your health is to develop all four.

A powerful synergy exists between these different components of fitness. For instance, cardiovascular fitness is known as the best way to decrease your risk of heart disease and high blood pressure, while strength training is an important way to reduce your risk of osteoporosis. But as we study the women who perform cardiovascular exercise like brisk walking, we realize it has a positive impact on bone strength as well as heart health. Recent studies have shown that, in addition to being good for bones, strength training seems to reduce the risk of heart disease by lowering blood pressure and cholesterol levels. And we realize today that weight loss is best achieved through a mix of cardiovascular and strength training exercises.

FITNESS AT ANY AGE

You are never too young or too old to benefit from becoming physically fit. Some of the benefits of exercise are gained almost immediately, while others become apparent years later. For instance, although we tend to think of osteoporosis as a disease that affects older women, your chance of developing it depends a great deal on the choices you make while you're young, because peak bone mass is built in the first three decades of life. Young girls who exercise appropriately build greater levels of bone mass than those who do not, decreasing their risk of developing osteoporosis later in life. *Appropriately* is the key word here, because too much exercise can be as harmful as too little. Excessive exercise can actually lead to premature bone loss and osteoporosis at a young age (see the sections on overtraining in chapter 7 and the female athlete triad in chapter 10).

Additionally, there is evidence that beginning to exercise at a young age helps decrease lifetime risk of developing other diseases, including diabetes and high blood pressure. One intriguing study concluded that an average of four hours of activity per week, beginning at puberty, significantly reduces the risk of developing breast cancer, probably through the effect of exercise on fluctuating hormones. Fluctuations in hormones also cause the symptoms (like mood swings and irritability, hot flashes and sleep disturbances) associated with premenstrual syndrome (PMS) and perimenopause, respectively, many of which can be reduced by regular exercise. And you may be interested to know that, although hormones have many effects on the female body, they do not have a significant effect on exercise performance. Likewise, birth control pills do not affect athletic performance.

As young women age, they begin to see other ways that fitness improves their health and quality of life, not the least of which is weight control. This is especially true as women enter their child-bearing years, as exercise can help to prevent excessive weight gain during pregnancy and can help you get back to your pre-pregnancy weight. More important, research has concluded that exercise is not only safe in pregnancy, it provides extra health benefits to both mom and baby (see the section on a healthier pregnancy in chapter 3).

There is controversy surrounding the guidelines published in 1994 by the American College of Obstetricians and

Gynecologists (ACOG) regarding exercise in pregnancy, particularly the recommendation that pregnant women should avoid most activities other than stationary biking and swimming. It is very important to realize that this recommendation was based on the *possibility* of risk to the fetus rather than on any evidence that other activities are detrimental. Some researchers have shown that women can participate in a variety of activities while pregnant, including running and light to moderate strength training with machines, without any harm to the fetus. Some activities, like scuba diving and exercise at high altitude, are generally not considered by anyone to be safe in pregnancy. After the first trimester, a pregnant woman should also avoid lying on her back during exercise, as this puts pressure on the large blood vessel that supplies blood to the uterus and fetus.

Additionally, ACOG recommends exercise at a lower level of intensity while pregnant, another recommendation that some experts feel is too conservative. Because every woman and every pregnancy is unique, it's important that you check with your doctor to see what's right for you.

Remaining active throughout the perimenopausal and postmenopausal years has tremendous health benefits as well. It's encouraging to know that although athletic performance starts to decline after age forty-five to fifty, this decline is gradual and relatively modest. Researchers have found evidence that continued physical activity reduces many of the common signs and symptoms associated with aging, including weight gain, sleep disturbances, and anxiety. In addition, staying active provides an important boost to many of your aging tissues, including the entire immune system. One more benefit of exercise seems to persist throughout the active woman's lifetime: researchers have found that fit women report better sex. This is presumed to be due to a variety of factors, including heightened sexual responses from enhanced blood flow and a boost in self-esteem.

GETTING STARTED ON THE PATH TO FITNESS

Although every woman's exercise program should be personalized, I generally recommend that most women begin a fitness program with cardiovascular exercise. This is because, of the four components of fitness, it's the one with the largest, quickest impact on your health. It is also the least intimidating, because most of us already know how to do some form of cardiovascular exercise. Cardiovascular, or *aerobic,* which means "using oxygen," is the type of exercise that "gets your blood pumping," like brisk walking, jogging, swimming, bicycling, and dancing. It improves your health in a variety of ways, including strengthening your heart and lowering your blood pressure. Ideally, simple flexibility exercises (i.e., stretching) are quickly incorporated into a cardiovascular exercise program, because they can help improve joint range of motion and reduce muscle tightness, which can make your new activity seem both more enjoyable and easier.

I recommend that most beginners spend four to six weeks getting comfortable with cardiovascular and flexibility exercises before adding strength training. Let me stress that this is not a magic formula, but from my experience with a number of patients, it seems to work. Spending a few weeks focusing on cardiovascular exercise allows you to develop a fitness base that you can then build upon. Perhaps most important, it gives you a chance to master one component of fitness, giving you the confidence to tackle another. Of course, if you are reading this and are already active, you may want to jump ahead to chapter 5, which discusses strength training. Or, if you have a medical condition such as arthritis that makes cardiovascular exercise difficult, you may also choose to start with strength training. Remember, this is *your* health and your fitness program. There are no exercises you *must* perform and there is no magic order in which exercises should be done.

The following chapters will explain the health impact of each of the components of fitness, and outline the framework of a complete exercise program. Based on what you discovered in this chapter about your own goals, you can choose where to focus your efforts to get the results *you* want. I always tell patients that beginning an exercise program is just like going into a restaurant. When you get there, a lot of factors may influence what you choose to eat. If you're trying to lose weight, you may search out the low-calorie choices; if you're watching your cholesterol, you may pick the fish over the steak. Or if you're just out to have a good time, you may want to try one of everything! You can think of fitness options in the same way, but instead of choosing among appetizers, entrées, and desserts, you're selecting among cardiovascular, flexibility, and strengthening exercise options. You can pick and choose among them as stepping-stones on your pathway to better health.

PART 2

THE BUILDING BLOCKS OF FITNESS

CHAPTER 3

THE HEART OF HEALTH: CARDIOVASCULAR FITNESS

Lynne, a bubbly thirty-five-year-old social worker, lost both of her parents to heart disease at a young age. She was worried about her own health because she had inherited a tendency toward high blood pressure and had very high cholesterol. Determined to reduce her risk of a heart attack, she began going to a gym, where she rode a stationary bike and jogged on a treadmill. After six months, her blood pressure had normalized and her cholesterol had dropped thirty points. Lynne said exercise worked "like magic."

WHAT HAPPENED TO LYNNE'S BLOOD PRESSURE and cholesterol levels may have seemed magical to her, but it's a phenomenon doctors see routinely. Through regular exercise, the heart (cardio) and blood vessels (vascular) get strong and healthy, a condition known as *cardiovascular fitness*. (You also may see this referred to as *cardiorespiratory fitness*, with "respiratory" referring to the lungs.) To understand how cardiovascular fitness lays the foundation for good health, it helps to have an understanding of how this amazing system works.

THE BODY'S PACKAGE-DELIVERY SYSTEM

I think of the cardiovascular system as the body's very own package-delivery service. Its primary job is to transport oxygen and other nutrients to the rest of the body. The heart serves as a main dispatch terminal, where red blood cells go to pick up "packages" of oxygen, which have arrived via the lungs. The heart then pumps the oxygen-filled blood cells out through a main "highway," the aorta. From there, the blood cells are diverted into hundreds of different areas of the body, traveling along blood vessels that vary in size (think smaller highways, country roads, city streets, and tiny avenues).

In some people, the blood cells race along like expensive sports cars, delivering their cargo quickly and efficiently before heading back to the heart for the next assignment. But in other people, blood cells have problems reaching their destinations. This is frequently the result of "traffic congestion" in blood vessels that have become narrowed by a buildup of cholesterol, a naturally occurring substance that's both produced by the liver and common to many foods we eat. The result of this slowdown is that the poor working tissue on the other side of this traffic snarl begins to run out of oxygen and energy. The exhausted tissue begins to slow down, makes more mistakes, and anxiously signals its growing distress if the much-needed oxygen doesn't arrive soon. Initially, you may not be aware of this drama unfolding within your body, but as the situation worsens, you may begin to interpret the body's distress signals as weakness, shortness of breath, or pain.

The heart itself is especially vulnerable to a delay in the arrival of oxygen. About the size of a fist, the heart is the most important muscle in your body. Unlike the majority of our other muscles, it is never able to take even a short break from working! It has its own dedicated blood vessels, called coronary arteries, which keep it supplied with oxygen. If the coronary arteries become clogged with cholesterol and the working heart muscle doesn't get enough oxygen, it is unable to continue functioning properly. This causes chest pain, known as *angina,* and often signals an impending heart attack.

Unfortunately for women, recent research suggests that women with cardiovascular disease are less likely to develop the typical symptoms of angina, and are more likely to experience vague symptoms like fatigue. For some women, this means that by the time cardiovascular disease becomes obvious, it may be too late. Two and a half million American women are hospitalized for heart disease every year, and one out of every five of them die, making heart disease the leading cause of death among women. Our lifestyle choices—like smoking, eating high-fat diets, and avoiding exercise—are often to blame. The simple choices you make every day, like taking the stairs or walking to the store, can ultimately play a role in whether or not you die from heart disease.

HOW CARDIOVASCULAR EXERCISE AFFECTS THE HEART

We know without a doubt that regular exercise makes the heart stronger and less susceptible to disease. There are several complex scientific theories as to why this is so. Just like any other muscle in the body, the heart muscle adapts to exercise by becoming stronger. Each heartbeat, or *pulse,* is simply a result of contraction of the heart muscle. The stronger the muscle, the stronger the contraction.

Now, remember, with each beat of the heart, blood cells are being sent to deliver those packages of oxygen and other nutrients that the body needs. When the heart muscle is stronger, the heart becomes more efficient at delivering the needed goods. All the hardworking tissues of your body, from your brain to your kidneys to the muscles in your arms and legs, benefit from this. And the heart itself receives a special benefit from this improved efficiency: it takes fewer heartbeats per minute to deliver the oxygen and nutrients the body needs. This means the "pump" itself gets a break and doesn't have to work quite as hard, which will help it to stay strong and healthy longer.

Amazingly, while the health benefit of strengthening your heart and reducing your heart rate is enormous, it takes only four to six weeks of regular exercise to achieve. One recent study found that women who simply walked for a total of *one hour each week* had a lower risk of heart attack. (Some of the other benefits of exercise, like improved sleep and stress reduction, can begin to occur immediately.) Of course, the reverse is also true. Once you stop exercising, you lose most of the benefits you just gained, which is why it's so important to put together an exercise program that you can stick with.

The heart has been called a "female organ" when it comes to emotional matters. I tell some of my busy female patients who say they can't find time to exercise that the heart truly *is* a "female organ," because like them, it never takes a break. I encourage them to think about how they feel when they are constantly pressured to get things done without enough support or help. That's not a very pleasant feeling, but it is precisely the kind of pressure you subject your own heart to when you deny it the benefit provided by exercise.

THE ROLE OF OXYGEN

What do folding the laundry and running a marathon have in common?

They both require your body to respond to a demand for energy. No matter what activity you're engaged in, your body must provide enough energy to accomplish your mission. It does this through a series of chemical reactions, many of which require oxygen and are called *aerobic.* Your body can't store much oxygen, so it's critical that your body be able to transport and deliver it upon demand. If oxygen can't get to the cells that need it, the cells try to function without it (so called *anaerobic* activity). Unfortunately, they can't work for long without a supply of oxygen, and if it doesn't get there soon, the cells give up, stop working, and eventually die.

HOW CARDIOVASCULAR EXERCISE AFFECTS BLOOD PRESSURE

Blood pressure is the amount of force (i.e., pressure) generated in the arteries as your blood circulates throughout your body. Blood pressure patterns are unique to every individual, and can vary significantly throughout the course of a day. In fact, your blood pressure can go up or down by several points from minute to minute. Blood pressure is affected by a tremendous number of factors, including your level of activity, anxiety, caffeine, cigarette smoking, weight, and heredity. Many medications can also affect your blood pressure, including several over-the-counter cold medicines and weight-loss aids, primarily because they contain stimulants.

Many people know that blood pressure is expressed as a ratio of two numbers, and quite a few even know that anything above 140/90 is considered high. But what exactly do those numbers mean?

Blood pressure = systolic pressure/diastolic pressure

The systolic pressure, or top number, is the pressure generated by the heart's contraction when it pumps blood out into the arteries. The diastolic pressure, or bottom number, is the pressure maintained on the walls of the arteries between heartbeats. If either of these numbers is high, damage to the heart and blood vessels can result.

In the past, doctors thought that exercise helped to lower blood pressure simply by contributing to weight loss. Now we know that a regular exercise program can lower blood pressure *independent* of weight loss. We still don't know exactly how this happens. Most likely, it is because exercise suppresses levels of certain hormones (like adrenaline) that elevate blood pressure. Whatever the mechanism, multiple studies have shown that we can easily drop both the systolic and diastolic (top and bottom) components of blood pressure 5 to 10 points with exercise alone. Some of my patients have been successful enough at lowering blood pressure through exercise that they have been able to stop taking antihypertensive medications, saving them money and the risk of medication side effects.

And just like a reduction in heart rate, the lowering of blood pressure can be seen in as little as four weeks of regular cardiovascular exercise.

HOW CARDIOVASCULAR EXERCISE AFFECTS CHOLESTEROL

Just as it can produce a positive effect on blood pressure, exercise also works to improve one's cholesterol, or lipid, profile, by lowering total cholesterol, and increasing HDL cholesterol (the so-called good cholesterol). Why is it important to lower our total cholesterol? It helps to understand that cholesterol is a normal substance in our bodies, produced by the liver and used for such important tasks as building hormones. But the liver is quite capable of making most if not all of the cholesterol we need, so most of the cholesterol in the foods we eat is not useful to the body.

We get rid of this extra cholesterol by transporting it through the body in a "package" called a *lipoprotein*. Lipoprotein packages come in various sizes, including the low-density, or LDL, and the high-density, or HDL, varieties. LDLs transport cholesterol throughout the body, but often leaves some cholesterol sticking to the walls of the blood vessels. This buildup of cholesterol, or *plaques,* on the blood vessel walls is commonly known as hardening of the arteries, and increases the risk of heart attack or stroke. HDLs, on the other hand, whisk cholesterol out of the bloodstream by transporting it to the liver, where it can be recycled into bile salts and excreted. Because high levels of HDL reduce the amount of cholesterol in circulation, they are associated with lower risk of heart disease. Estrogen really helps women out here, because it encourages the production of HDLs over LDLs. Exercise provides the same advantage, apparently by stimulating the production of an enzyme called lipoprotein lipase, which also encourages the production of HDLs over LDLs. The end result? Less cholesterol gets stuck behind in the arteries, and our risk of cardiovascular disease drops.

For years, doctors believed estrogen helped prevent heart disease. Studies showed that it helps keep blood vessels more supple, decreasing risk of high blood pressure. It raises HDL cholesterol (the good one) and lowers LDL cholesterol (the bad one). And it was reported to decrease risk of a heart attack by up to 50 percent. But now, the glow of estrogen is fading. Recent studies show that it is not the magic bullet it was believed to be, and that estrogen supplements may not prevent heart disease after all. However, unlike estrogen, exercise *has been shown* to prevent heart disease. Currently, we believe that this is due to a combination of the positive effects of exercise mentioned earlier, such as lowered blood pressure and cholesterol levels, and improved efficiency of the cardiovascular system. However, there are several exciting theories that may prove to be equally important. For instance, the body appears to have an "angry" immune response to cholesterol plaques being deposited in arterial walls. Unfortunately, such a reaction can cause further damage to the blood vessel walls. Some researchers believe that exercise's protective effect against heart disease has to do with its special ability to dampen this immune response.

So remember, although we don't know all the hows and whys, we already know that exercise is one of the answers. As doctors continue looking for a magic pill to ward off heart disease, you can make exercise your own magic pill.

OTHER HEALTH BENEFITS OF CARDIOVASCULAR EXERCISE

Helps Control Diabetes

Diabetes, a disease that affects over 135 million people worldwide, is growing at alarming rates in industrialized countries like the United States, and is frequently associated with obesity and sedentary lifestyles. It is characterized by high levels of glucose (or sugar) in the bloodstream. Those with diabetes have an increased risk of developing many serious illnesses, like heart disease, stroke, and kidney failure. This is because too much glucose in the bloodstream results in damage to blood vessel walls, preventing the delivery of oxygen and other important nutrients to the body's hard-working organs, such as the heart, brain, and kidneys.

Many people mistakenly believe diabetes is simply the result of eating sugary foods. In reality, all forms of carbohydrate, including bread, fruits, and vegetables, are broken down into glucose, which the body relies on for energy. Glucose can be used immediately for energy, or stored in muscles or fat for later use. Insulin, a hormone produced by the pancreas, helps regulate the use and storage of glucose.

The most common type of diabetes, called type 2 diabetes, is often associated with obesity. When there is too much glucose around (often from overeating), the pancreas is forced to produce more insulin to help get all the extra glucose into storage in muscle and fat cells. These higher levels of insulin circulating in the bloodstream can lead to plaque formation in the blood vessels, and seems to encourage fat storage in the abdomen (known as the "apple" pattern), which is associated with increased risk of heart disease. As the insulin continues to push glucose into muscle and fat cells, the overstuffed cells rebel. They fight back by becoming "resistant" to insulin. This resistance results in less glucose getting into cells, and more staying in the circulation. But the higher level of glucose in the bloodstream is dangerous, so the pancreas is ordered to produce more insulin. This goes on until, eventually, the pancreas isn't able to keep up with the demand to produce more and more insulin. Insulin production begins to fall off, leaving the glucose floating in the bloodstream, resulting in the diagnosis of diabetes.

How does cardiovascular exercise help? Exercise uses up the glucose that's stored in the muscle cells. This makes the muscles hungry for more glucose, so they stop being resistant when insulin pushes more glucose into the muscle. This decrease in resistance to insulin breaks the cycle of increasing insulin and glucose levels in the bloodstream, and prevents the blood vessel damage that occurs from high amounts of glucose and insulin staying in circulation. If exercise is regular enough to use up some of the body's fat stores, the whole body becomes more sensitive to insulin. The net result is that your pancreas needs to produce less insulin, glucose gets used immediately for energy or is stored efficiently for later use, and your blood vessels stay clean and healthy.

History indicates that as early as 600 B.C., exercise was recommended as treatment for diabetes. Despite extensive research and development of new, state-of-the-art medications, exercise is still proving to be one of the most effective treatments in the battle against this common disease. The ongoing Nurses' Health Study recently found that women with type 2 diabetes who exercise moderately or vigorously for four hours each week have a 40 percent lower risk of cardiovascular disease than women who don't exercise. Even strolling at a leisurely pace (less than 2 mph) for forty-five minutes a day was found to lower a diabetic woman's risk of cardiovascular disease.

Stimulates the Immune System

The human immune system is one of nature's most fascinating networks: it functions as your body's own "spy" organization, complete with several of its own versions of James Bond. Its many components include the spleen, lymph nodes, bone marrow, and thousands of microscopic cells circulating through the bloodstream, all under the influence of a variety of hormones. The immune system is responsible for tracking down and killing invading infectious agents like viruses and bacteria, as well as for ferreting out and fighting cancer cells. Exercise seems to stimulate increased activity by at least some of the components of the immune system, and has been reported to decrease the risk of everything from the common cold to colon cancer.

How does this happen? As we age, the immune system tends to decline in power. But studies of older women show that exercise seems to give it a boost. Women who exercise were found to have more active "killer cells" circulating through their bloodstreams, seeking out unwelcome invaders. And some researchers theorize that the increase in heart rate during exercise sends more of these cells surging into the bloodstream.

Improves Mental Health

Regular physical activity also improves mental health. Studies have shown that in addition to improving psychological well-being and boosting self-esteem, exercise reduces the symptoms of depression, anxiety, and panic disorder.

We don't understand all the ways exercise works to improve mental health, but it's believed to be due to a combination of psychological, biological, and social mechanisms. Researchers have found that ten minutes of moderate aerobic exercise lifts mood and also decreases feelings of fatigue. Additionally, some studies have shown a tantalizing effect on other psychological functioning. One study showed a decrease in confusion with ten to twenty minutes of exercise, which could have important implications in preserving mental function with aging.

Results in Healthier Pregnancy

A century ago, doctors treated pregnant women as though they were extremely fragile. It was believed that physical exertion caused infertility, miscarriages, premature labor, and fetal malformations. Today, however, the evidence is mounting that exercise is one of the smartest moves a pregnant woman can make.

Dr. James F. Clapp III, a leading authority in the study of exercise during pregnancy, has found that vigorous exercise has positive effects on the health of both moms and babies. For instance, regular, vigorous weight-bearing exercise, like running and aerobics, doesn't increase risk of premature births and is associated with shorter labors, fewer complications, and reduced need for medical interventions at the time of delivery. Additionally, women who exercise vigorously have babies with a little less body fat than the average. This is thought to be a great asset in helping to ward off obesity later in life, which is especially important given the fact that obesity among children in the United States is currently at an all-time high. Recent studies suggest one other advantage for babies born to exercising moms: They may be smarter. Dr. Clapp found that five-year-olds whose mothers exercised during pregnancy had higher scores on standardized intelligence tests.

Even though recent research suggests that maximum benefits are obtained when the exercise is vigorous, numerous studies have concluded that *any* regular exercise program is beneficial in reducing pregnancy-associated musculoskeletal complaints like back pain. It also improves body image and decreases weight gain and fat deposition in late pregnancy. Of course, pregnant women need to check with their doctors for any exercise limitations based on their individual pregnancies.

Even if, for whatever reasons, you didn't exercise during your pregnancy, exercising *after* delivery has benefits, too. It's associated with lower levels of stress and depression, and increases the likelihood that you will get back to your prepregnancy weight.

CARDIOVASCULAR FITNESS LAYS THE FOUNDATION FOR GOOD HEALTH

In summary, cardiovascular exercise strengthens the heart and lowers blood pressure and cholesterol levels, thereby reducing the risk of heart disease and stroke. It stimulates your immune system, helps control diabetes, reduces anxiety and depression, and makes pregnancy healthier. Still not enough to convince you to get moving? There's more. Every day, it seems, we find new ways that cardiovascular fitness enhances a woman's health. Weight-bearing cardiovascular exercises like walking reduce osteoporosis. Non- or low-impact cardiovascular exercises like swimming and bicycling help patients with osteoarthritis. And any exercise at all seems to have a positive impact on weight control, depression, and anxiety.

Unfortunately, every year there are stories of people who suddenly suffer a heart attack during exertion, like a game of tennis, or jogging, or shoveling snow. It is important to realize that although their heart attacks occurred during a

IMPORTANT RISK FACTORS FOR HEART DISEASE

Family history (genetic predisposition)

High cholesterol (high LDL/low HDL)

High blood pressure

Diabetes

Obesity

Smoking

Did you notice that only one of these risk factors is beyond your control? (Hint: We don't choose our families!) But each of these other factors can be directly or indirectly impacted by exercise. Yes, even smoking, because many smokers finally quit when they begin exercising. And although you can't change your genes, you may be able to alter the future course of your family history by improving your own health through exercise and by being a positive role model for your spouse and children. Studies have shown that although more and more children in the United States are sedentary and overweight, they are more likely to exercise if one or both parents also exercise. Although there is no denying the strong genetic component of heart disease, the risks imposed by lifestyle factors are *at least* as important.

period of exertion, exercise itself didn't cause the problem, underlying heart disease did. *This is why it is so important to see your doctor before beginning an exercise program.* Your doctor will evaluate your individual risk factors for heart disease and determine whether you already have underlying heart disease, which may require that you modify your exercise plan. The American College of Sports Medicine recommends a screening exercise treadmill test for all women over fifty—or younger, if they have known risk factors for heart disease—before they begin an exercise program. This continues to be an area of controversy, especially because women are more likely to have a false-positive test (meaning you don't have heart disease but the test falsely indicates that you do). The bottom line? Talk with your doctor about what's right for *you.*

DESIGNING YOUR CARDIOVASCULAR FITNESS PROGRAM

Ready to get started on your way to a healthier heart? Let's begin by assessing your current level of cardiovascular fitness. We will use a very simple test that you can do at home, with a friend or by yourself. (Note: There are more sophisticated and formal ways to measure fitness, including a treadmill test performed by a health professional. If you would like to have a formal assessment done, check with your doctor.) As previously mentioned, it is a good idea for every woman to have a health assessment by her doctor before beginning any exercise program.

For this simple test, all you will need is comfortable clothing, a pair of walking or running shoes, and a watch or a stopwatch. Choose a flat surface, set your watch, and start moving. The goal is to cover as much ground as you can in ten minutes. If you are already fit, you may be able to jog or even run for the full ten minutes. If you are a bona fide couch potato, you may not be able to walk more than a few minutes without needing to take a break, which is okay. *Do not berate yourself for what you can't do—congratulate yourself for what you can do.* If you feel you didn't do well on the initial assessment, take heart: The worse shape you are in initially, the faster you will progress. Also, it might encourage you to know that multiple studies suggest that the greatest decrease in risk for heart disease is seen when sedentary people become moderately active. This means that you don't have to increase your activity to the level of a marathon runner to reap the greatest heart-healthy benefits of exercise.

Some women will feel more challenged to improve their health if they know how they compare to others; for some, comparisons to others is intimidating or discouraging. If you are in the former category, measure the distance you were able to cover. You can do this with a *pedometer,* a small device that clips onto your shoe or waistband, costs about $25, and records the distance you walk or jog. Or you may choose to drive along your course to check its length. If you covered more than a mile, you are significantly more fit than the average woman. You should still follow the principles outlined in this section, but you will be able to progress more rapidly.

For those who don't want to compare themselves to others, it's perfectly okay to use "landmarks" like certain trees, fence posts, or buildings instead of recording actual mileage. Whatever method you choose, write down the results of your first assessment. This is the starting point against which you will measure your progress.

MAPPING YOUR PLAN

Imagine you are beginning a trip that will involve driving across a country you've never visited before. You would probably plan at least part of your trip in advance, thinking about your budget, time constraints, and the points of interest you don't want to miss. Beginning an exercise program is similar to planning such a trip: it makes a lot of sense to gather information and then plan your own exercise program, rather than just jumping in and hoping it will all work out. The steps you took in the first section were designed to help you identify both your starting point and your goals, and to plan for such issues as budget and time constraints. Now it's time to design your trip's itinerary: your personal fitness program. We'll do that by applying five fitness factors.

FIVE FITNESS FACTORS

1. Type of Activity

The *type* of activity you choose can be anything that uses your large muscle groups (especially your legs) in a continuous, rhythmic motion. This can include walking, jogging, dancing, skipping rope, or playing a vigorous set of tennis. It's important to emphasize continuous. Contrary to what one might think, some activities do not really improve cardiovascular health. For instance, standing in the outfield during a softball game or playing a leisurely game of badminton may be fun, but it won't give your heart enough of a workout to provide much health benefit.

Although any activity that gets you moving is fine, beginners should avoid choosing as an initial activity any exercise that involves using unfamiliar equipment (such as the stair stepper, ski machine, or rowing ergometer). I say this for two reasons: because using unfamiliar equipment raises the possibility of injury, especially when one's fitness base is still small; and unfamiliar equipment can be intimidating, making you lose confidence in your ability to succeed at exercise. After the first several weeks, when you're confident in your exercise abilities, you'll want to add new activities (see fitness factor 5).

Choosing Your Initial Activity

Remember, cardiovascular exercise, also known as aerobic exercise, is continuous movement, the type that gets your heart pumping more quickly and your breath coming a bit faster.

Some Activities for Improving Cardiovascular Fitness:

Walking	Running
Bicycling	Swimming
Rowing	Stair climbing
Dancing	Skating
Hiking	Cross-country skiing
Jumping rope	

Any activity that you choose will have a beneficial effect on your heart's health. However, the personal exercise history questionnaire and individual health goals identified in chapter 1 should help you to hone in on an activity that may be the best fit for you. For instance, if osteoporosis is a concern for you, then you may want to choose a *weight-bearing* activity like walking rather than a non-weight-bearing activity like swimming, as walking has been shown to have a positive impact on bone density.

What exactly is "weight-bearing" exercise?
Weight-bearing exercise is a term that creates confusion for a lot of women. This term entered our daily language when doctors began to realize that exercises requiring a woman to bear her own weight were superior for improving bone density and decreasing the risk of osteoporosis. Some women confuse "weight-bearing" with "impact." An exercise can be high-impact, such as running; lower impact, such as walking; or non-impact, such as cross-country skiing. However, all of these are weight-bearing activities, and all of them are good for the bones. In contrast, swimming is a non-weight-bearing activity (because the water does the weight-bearingn work for us). Swimming can be a great way to improve cardiovascular health and is easy on the joints, but it won't give you the bone-boosting benefits of a weight-bearing activity.

When choosing your first activity, consider the following:

Consideration	Possible Choice:
You haven't been active in the past year.	Any activity you already know how to do, and preferably one that's easy on the joints. Examples: walking, swimming, stationary bicycling.

Consideration	Possible Choice:
Osteoporosis prevention is a concern.	A weight-bearing activity over a non-weight-bearing activity. Examples: walking, jogging, dancing instead of swimming or stationary bicycling.
Your goal is weight loss.	Any activity that you can work up to sustaining for an hour. Examples: walking, bicycling, swimming, jogging.
You plan to exercise at home.	Walking or fitness videotapes; consider swimming or bicycling if you already have a pool or stationary bike.
You want to exercise with a partner.	Walking, dancing, taking aerobic classes at a gym.
You have hip or knee pain.	Swimming; see a doctor for diagnosis and treatment of the hip/knee pain.
You have shoulder pain.	Walking; see a doctor for diagnosis and treatment of the shoulder pain.

Start Off Slowly

It's a good idea to spend a few minutes warming up at the beginning of your exercise session. Do this by beginning your activity at a leisurely pace, and then increasing your intensity after five to ten minutes. This warm-up stimulates blood flow to the muscles you'll be using, delivering those nutrients and oxygen your working muscles will need. Similarly, a few minutes of cooling down allows your heart rate to gradually return to normal. Make sure to slow your pace and continue moving for a few minutes after your workout until your heart rate comes down. Stopping exercise suddenly can make your heart rate drop more quickly, leaving you feeling light-headed or dizzy.

CHOOSING AN EXERCISE VIDEO

Exercising at home with a video exercise tape is popular among women and can be a very effective, time-efficient workout. Finding an exercise video that is right for you requires a little sleuthing. Look for videos in which instructors give alignment tips, provide easier alternatives for difficult moves, and perform a wide variety of different exercises. A terrific resource is Collage Video's guide to exercise videos, 800-433-6769 or *www.collagevideo.com.*

A word of warning: A common practice is to take a previously released tape, repackage it with a new cover and other cosmetic changes, and sell it as a "new" tape. The video experts at Collage can tell you if this is the case with a new video you're thinking about buying.

2. Intensity of Exercise

For many women who have not exercised on a regular basis, walking is a great activity. In fact, walking is the single most popular form of all aerobic activities, largely because essentially everyone already knows how to do it. However, not everyone understands the difference between walking *for locomotion* and walking *to develop fitness.* This is where the next fitness factor, *intensity,* becomes important. A casual stroll may be relaxing, but unless you increase your pace, your heart won't get much benefit. However, you also needn't sprint along at breakneck speed. No matter what activity you choose, you need to find an intensity level in the middle ground—not too fast, but not too slow. Fortunately, this is easy to do by using one of the following techniques.

Measure Your Heart Rate

Since we are trying to develop heart health, a great way to measure success is by monitoring heart rate. No, it's not necessary to buy a fancy gizmo to do this. All it takes is a watch with a second hand, and a little practice locating your pulse. (Although if you *want* to buy a fancy gizmo, a heart-rate monitor will do the work for you.) To begin, find the radial pulse at your wrist, or the carotid pulse at your neck. Locate your radial pulse by turning your left hand palm up and placing the tip of your second and third fingers on your wrist near the base of your thumb. Find your carotid pulse by slipping the fingertips upward from your Adam's apple and then sideways, away from your windpipe. You'll find the carotid pulse here, beneath the line of your jaw.

You may have to apply light pressure to feel the pulse; don't press too hard, or you will actually occlude the pulse. You may find it easier to locate your pulse if you move around briskly for a few minutes first (feeling that your heart is beating just a bit harder makes the pulsation stronger and easier to detect). When you have located the pulse, you will feel its rhythmic beat under your fingertips.

Using a watch or clock with a second hand (or, even easier, a digital watch), begin counting the number of beats. The goal is to figure out how many times your heart is beating per minute. This number is called your *resting heart rate*. You can do this by counting each beat for a full sixty seconds, or you can get a quick estimate by counting for ten seconds and multiplying that number by six, or by counting for fifteen seconds and multiplying by four. An average resting heart rate for a healthy woman is usually between sixty and ninety beats per minute, but this number can be affected by a wide variety of factors, including many medications (such as diet pills, cold preparations, and some blood pressure medications), anxiety, and dehydration.

Now that you are comfortable finding your resting heart rate, try taking your heart rate after you've exercised vigorously for a few minutes. Your pulse should be even easier to find, although it may take a bit of practice to find and count your heart rate while moving. As soon as you begin to slow down or stop exercise, your heart rate will also begin to fall. For this reason, I generally recommend using the ten-second-count method.

The faster your heart is beating, the more quickly oxygen is being supplied to your muscles. There is a point at which no matter how much oxygen your working muscles demand, your heart can't pump any harder (or faster) to make the delivery. This point is called your *maximum heart rate (MHR)*. How do you know what your maximum heart rate is? A doctor can perform a special type of exercise stress test to determine precisely what your MHR is, but most people can use a simple formula to estimate their maximum heart rate:

220 − your age in years = MHR

So, if you are forty years old, your estimated MHR is 220 − 40, or 180 beats/minute. There is some controversy about how reliable this method is, but I have found that it holds up as a pretty good estimate, especially for people who aren't already active. If you are a regular exerciser already, your MHR is probably a bit higher, because your heart is able to work harder upon demand. If you fall into this group, you might want to use the following formula instead:

210 − half your age in years = MHR

So, if you are a regular exerciser who is forty years old, your estimated MHR is 210 − 20, or 190 beats/minute. One caveat, however. This latter formula was developed initially by studying male athletes. It doesn't seem to have been studied much in women, but I have several patients who think it works well for them.

You may be relieved to know that you only have to raise your heart rate to a portion of your MHR to see health benefits from exercise. This is called the *target heart rate (THR)*, the number of heartbeats per minute that will allow you to achieve cardiovascular fitness. If you are a beginner, aim for exercise intensity that increases your heart rate to 60 to 70 percent of your MHR.

HEART-RATE MONITORS

Once a tool of elite athletes, heart-rate monitors are now used by a wide variety of athletes at a wide variety of levels. Particularly popular with runners, walkers, and triathletes, the traditional model, which includes a strap worn around the chest, transmits your heart rate to a monitor worn like a wristwatch. Watch for a variety of new models that are beginning to hit the market, like the one that fits on the finger of a swimmer. You can buy one with lots of bells and whistles (which costs upward of $150), or the most simple version for as little as $50.

Polar is a good brand of heart-rate monitor to look for, as the company has a variety of different styles available and has years of experience behind their products. Polar also makes a sports bra with a specially designed pocket that a monitor fits in, eliminating the need for an extra chest strap. This is a particularly popular option with many of my patients who are runners.

THR = between 60 and 70 percent of MHR

For our forty-year-old beginning exerciser, the MHR was 180 beats/minute. Sixty percent of 180 is 108 beats/minute, 70 percent of 180 is 126 beats/minute. Therefore, the THR range for this beginning exerciser is between 108 and 126 beats/minute. You can check the chart below for your own THR.

What does it mean if our model exerciser's heart rate is staying below 108 beats/minute? It probably means that she's not working her heart hard enough to get the best benefits from her exercise. If she's much over 126 beats/minute, she's probably working her heart too hard to be able to keep up at that intensity for long. That means that she's more likely to feel winded or tired before long, and will have to

Target Heart Rate Chart

Age	MHR	60%	70%	85%
20	200	120	140	170
25	195	117	137	166
30	190	114	133	162
35	185	111	130	157
40	180	108	126	153
45	175	105	123	149
50	170	102	119	145
55	165	99	116	140
60	160	96	112	136
65	155	93	109	132
70	150	90	105	128
75	145	87	102	123

slow down or quit exercising. *This is why* measuring intensity is so important, especially for beginners: If you're pushing your heart faster than it's ready to go, the experience of exercise will most likely be an unpleasant one, and you're more likely to get discouraged and quit. Conversely, if you're not getting your heart rate up to 60 percent of your MHR, you won't get the results you want to see. Exercising at an appropriate intensity allows you to achieve your fitness and health goals.

Above is a chart that gives you a range of THRs for a variety of ages. However, for anyone who's not a math equation lover, I recommend finding and memorizing the ten-second range that corresponds with your desired THR. For instance, our forty-year-old beginner has a THR of 108 to 126 beats per minute. If she counts her pulse for just ten seconds, then multiplies that number by six, she'll be able to see if she is exercising in her THR. But to make it easy, she can figure out in advance that 18 to 21 beats in ten seconds corresponds with her THR range of 108 to 126 beats per minute. So now, every time she exercises, she needs only to check her pulse for ten seconds to see if she's exercising at her desired intensity level.

While beginners should aim for 60 to 70 percent of their MHR, more experienced exercisers will want to push this up toward 85% of MHR for higher levels of cardiovascular training.

A final note: Measuring target heart rate is probably not appropriate for pregnant women who exercise, because of all the additional variables (like fetal activity) that affect heart rate during pregnancy. If you're pregnant, try the alternative method of measuring intensity, *rate of perceived exertion,* below.

HEART RATE AS A MEASURE OF SUCCESS

How quickly your heart rate slows down after exercise is a good indicator of how fit you are. The better shape your cardiovascular system is in, the faster your heart rate returns to normal when you stop exercising. A woman who is moderately fit can expect her heart rate to drop at least thirteen to fifteen beats/minute until it returns to baseline; a very fit woman will find it drops much more quickly. Watch for this to happen *to you* as you become more heart-healthy! If your heart rate drops twelve or fewer beats per minute, check with your doctor, because this could be a warning signal that you have heart disease.

Rate of Perceived Exertion—RPE (An Alternative to Measuring Heart Rate)

I recommend that you get in the habit of checking your own heart rate during exercise for two reasons. First, it is a simple way to keep in touch with your goal of improving your heart health; second, it serves as a reminder that you personally are in charge of what happens to it. However, it is important that you remember that the heart-rate formula is an *estimate*. There is some controversy among exercise scientists regarding whether or not heart-rate formulas are really accurate. If you have trouble with this method, find it distracting from your exercise session, or question its accuracy, I recommend using a rate of perceived exertion (RPE) scale. This type of scale is based on your own perception of how intense your exercise session feels. The most well known is the Borg Perceived Exertion scale, shown on the next page.

The Borg RPE Scale

6		14	
7	Very, very light	15	Hard
8		16	
9	Very light	17	Very hard
10		18	
11	Fairly light	19	Very, very hard
12		20	
13	Somewhat hard		

This scale seems to work pretty well for those who've memorized it, or for those gym goers who see it posted on the walls at their gym. The target for most people is 12 or 13. However, some women have complained to me that they can't keep these numbers in mind. Several have asked me for a scale that starts at 1, not 6, which is why I created the simple scale below.

An Alternate RPE Scale

1 Very, very easy
2 Very easy
3 Easy
4 Not so easy
5 Getting challenging
6 Challenging, but not too hard
7 Hard
8 Very hard
9 Very, very hard
10 Maximal effort . . . can't sustain it for long!

Since this is much less precise than measuring THR, you might be surprised to know that in exercise studies, RPE holds up pretty well as a way to estimate your exercise intensity level. Still, you must try to be honest with yourself if you choose to use this method of measuring progress. Staying in the lowest numbers on the scale will keep you below your THR, and you may fall short of your goals. Some general guidelines are as follows: You should find yourself able to carry on a conversation easily if you're at a RPE of 1 to 2; begin working up a sweat at 3 to 4; and still be able to speak but not in full sentences at 6 to 7. An RPE of 6 or 7 is a good target for beginners, while more experienced exercisers might push for 8 or even 9.

Try comparing the two methods (RPE and THR) to see what works best for you. Try checking your pulse when you feel you're at a RPE of 7. Generally, I'd expect you to be at about 70 to 75 percent of your THR. Remember, both THR and RPE are *estimates* designed to help you monitor your exercise intensity.

Will a lower-intensity workout help burn more fat than a higher-intensity one?
No. This common misconception is based on the fact that at lower intensity levels, we are able to use calories from fat more easily. This means that mathematically, the *percentage* of fat burned during low-intensity workouts is higher than the percentage burned during harder workouts. But the *total* number of calories burned is what really counts, and the harder you exercise, the more total calories you burn.

3 and 4. Duration and Frequency

The third and fourth fitness factors to take into account when designing your individual exercise program are *duration* and *frequency*. These refer to that elusive factor we all want more of: *time*. How much time you need to exercise to achieve your goals has become a topic of controversy over the past few years. When it comes to deciding how long to exercise, many of my patients are understandably confused about the current recommendations. For many years, doctors recommended a minimum of twenty to thirty minutes of vigorous activity at least three days a week. Recently, however, health and fitness experts like the Surgeon General, the Centers for Disease Control (CDC), and the American College of Sports Medicine (ACSM) have all begun to advocate that we can "accumulate" thirty minutes of exercise over a day (for instance, ten minutes of gardening and two ten-minute walks rather than exercising for thirty minutes consecutively). I suspect this recommendation is primarily to encourage the 85 percent of us who are not regularly active to get off our couches and move. One study even found that walking for as little as five minutes at a time, six times a day had a slightly positive effect on fitness.

The real answer to the question "How much exercise is enough?" depends on each individual woman's goals. To reduce stress and make some health gains, accumulating thirty minutes of activity over the course of a day is sufficient. If this strategy works to get you moving, then your health will certainly benefit. In other words, *anything* is better than *nothing*. But if weight loss is one of your goals, you should know that recent studies suggest that one longer (thirty-minute) exercise session is superior to accumulating several shorter ones. Other studies indicate that longer sessions also maximize the positive effect of exercise on heart disease.

I personally advocate viewing these new recommendations as the *minimum* amount of activity a healthy body needs, but not as a *maximum* goal. I still recommend twenty to sixty minutes of continuous exercise at least three days weekly for most women. In general, exercising three days a week will help you reach—and maintain—an acceptable level of fitness. If your goal is weight loss, three days a week will probably not be enough. For weight loss, aim for exercising five days a week. But not five consecutive days. Your body needs at least one day of rest. Heart health can be improved significantly in the shorter duration of exercise (twenty to thirty minutes); weight loss will require a longer session (thirty to sixty minutes). A good approach for some

---

Want to add more activity into your daily life? Try the following:

Walk a little more: Park an extra block or two away when running errands; take the stairs instead of the elevator or escalator; get out of the car instead of using drive-through windows.

Lose one convenient or automatic gadget: Hide the remote control; trade your electric mixer, can opener, or juicer for the manual kind; use pruning shears instead of an electric hedge trimmer.

Move at least once an hour, no matter what you're doing: Get on the floor and do sit-ups during TV commercial breaks; walk briskly to a coworker's office instead of sending an e-mail; take a two-minute stretch break from the computer.

---

of my patients has been thirty to forty-five minutes of continuous exercise three or four days a week, and accumulating thirty minutes of exercise through short walks on the other days.

5. Progression of Exercise Program

The final factor that needs to be considered in individualizing your exercise program is *progression*. (Learning how to continue to make progress your program is so important that part 3 of this book is dedicated to dealing with this fitness factor). Depending on your goals, you'll want to make periodic changes in your routine, such as adding different exercises, increasing speed, or adding hills to your walking program. Make these changes too quickly, and you increase your risk of injury; make them too slowly, and you miss some of the benefits you could be gaining. In general, I recommend progressing one and only one of the first four fitness factors every few weeks. Some possibilities to consider: Try a new machine at the gym or a different fitness tape or class, add five or ten minutes to your exercise session, or include a few minutes of exercise at a higher heart rate.

This may sound simple, but I've found that of the five fitness factors, progression is the one many of my patients tend to ignore. *However, ignoring the progression factor undoubtedly will prevent you from maximizing your health and fitness gains.* This is because the human body learns to adapt to repeated patterns of movement, and stops learning when no new information is presented. Think of it this way: Never progressing your fitness program would be like staying in first grade indefinitely, instead of learning a new, progressive curriculum with each passing year. Obviously, such monotonous repetition would get pretty boring, which is why lack of progression makes an exercise program much easier to quit. Progression helps you stay motivated as you continue to see health benefits while you conquer new exercise challenges.

WRITE IT DOWN

Many women, especially those who are novice exercisers, find that writing down their personal plan for fitness helps them stay focused and motivated. Keeping the five fitness factors in mind, complete the worksheet below. This will be Part One of your personal exercise program. Plan to follow it for the first four weeks, although remember, it is *your* exercise program: you can change any of the fitness factors at any time. Use the samples in the next few pages for inspiration, but use your knowledge of yourself to design a program that is realistic for you!

Part One of My Personal Exercise Program

Cardiovascular Fitness

Results of my first fitness assessment:

Activity I plan to start with:

Intensity level I'll try to maintain, and the way I'll monitor it:

Duration of each planned exercise session:

Frequency I plan to exercise (mark these days on your calendar!):

My plan for progression of my exercise program is:

My fitness goals include:

My health goals include:

To help stay motivated, I will:

SAMPLE EXERCISE PROGRAM FOR CARDIOVASCULAR FITNESS

#1: A Walking Program

I met Laurie when her mother, who became my patient, had a heart attack at the age of fifty-one. Laurie was a pleasant twenty-six-year-old moderately overweight schoolteacher who had her mother's smile and fondness for sweets. At her mother's insistence, Laurie came in for a general physical examination. Other than her weight and borderline-high cholesterol, Laurie was healthy. She was very interested in learning about healthy ways to control her weight and reduce her risk for heart disease. She completed a self-evaluation (like the one you did in part 1 of this book) and then began a walking program like the one outlined below. One year later, she was still walking five days a week, had lost seventeen pounds, and had a healthy cholesterol level.

Laurie's Personal Exercise Plan

Results of first fitness assessment: Laurie was pleased that she was able to walk without stopping for the entire ten minutes, but after five minutes of brisk walking, she felt out of breath and had to slow down. She estimated that she walked about half a mile.

Activity: Laurie chose walking as her initial activity.

Intensity level: Using the equation for target heart rate (THR), Laurie estimated her THR as 116 to 134. (220 − 26 = 194; 60 to 70 percent × 194 = 116 to 134 beats/minute). She began checking her heart rate while walking, aiming for a ten-second count of 20 beats (20 × 6 = 120), which put her in the middle of her target range.

Duration and frequency: Laurie began by walking twenty minutes every day after school.

To progress, Laurie added two minutes to her walks each week until she was walking for thirty minutes. She then started varying how intense her exercise sessions were by interspersing a few minutes of walking with her heart rate up to 155 (80 percent of her estimated maximum heart rate).

Laurie's first *fitness goal* was to be able to walk a mile in twenty minutes.

Her *health goals* were to decrease her risk of heart disease by lowering her cholesterol and weight.

To help stay motivated, Laurie kept two photos in her desk drawer at work. One was a picture she had taken of her mother

SAMPLE WALKING PROGRAM WEEKS 1 TO 4 (FOR A NOVICE EXERCISER)

Week One

Intensity: THR 60 percent; RPE score 4 to 6

Duration: twenty minutes (You can break this up into two ten-minute sessions. If you can't continue for ten minutes consecutively, just do the best you can but make sure your daily total is twenty minutes.)

Frequency: three to five days (Try not to walk all consecutive days, i.e., M, T, Th, Sat is better than M, T, W, Th.)

Begin and end each session with a slower pace to warm up and cool down

I also recommend ending each session with stretches for quadriceps, hamstrings, calves, and low back (see chapter 4 on flexibility).

Week Two

Intensity: THR 60 percent; RPE score 4 to 6

Duration: twenty-two to twenty-five minutes

Frequency: three to six days

Continue warm-up and cool-down and stretches

Week Three

Intensity: THR 60 to 70 percent; RPE score 5 to 7

Duration: twenty-five to thirty minutes

Frequency: four to six days

Continue warm-up and cool-down and stretches

Week Four

Intensity: THR 60 to 70 percent; RPE 5 to 7

Duration: thirty minutes

Frequency: four to six days

Continue warm-up and cool-down and stretches

in the hospital; the other was her favorite high school photo, taken when she was twenty pounds lighter. Whenever she thought about skipping her walk, she'd take out the pictures and remind herself why she had begun the walking program.

Like Laurie, many women choose walking as their first activity. Its many benefits include improved heart health and bone strength, and it aids in weight reduction and weight control. It is a great choice for almost anyone, although if you are very overweight you may find it too stressful on your back and the joints of your legs. If that sounds like you, consider sample program #2.

#2: A Pool Plan

Ronnie was a sunny thirty-seven-year-old mother of four who gained an extra fifteen pounds with each of her pregnancies. At 5'4'' and 196 pounds, she came in for evaluation of persistent knee pain. Ronnie's examination showed that she had poor flexibility of her knees and early degenerative arthritis. It was imperative that she lose weight to take some pressure off her knees, and she understood that diet alone was not the answer. She found a local YMCA with child care facilities and a pool. Ronnie began taking a water aerobics class as well as a half-hour stretching class. After a few weeks, when her knee pain decreased, she began riding the stationary bike to add variety to her workouts. Two years later she had lost almost all of what she gleefully referred to as "my baby fat."

Ronnie's Personal Exercise Plan

Results of first fitness assessment: Ronnie walked for only four minutes before she stopped, complaining of knee pain.

Activity: Initially intimidated by the idea of wearing a bathing suit, Ronnie visited the YMCA and was relieved to see a wide variety of women, from a pregnant woman to a grandmother with arthritis, taking a water aerobics class. She talked to a couple of the women, who were so friendly and inviting that she signed up for the next class. She also signed up for a beginner's stretching class.

Intensity level: Ronnie didn't want to count her heart rate, so she planned to try for a level of 6 to 7 on the RPE scale.

Duration: Although each class lasted forty-five minutes, Ronnie's first goal was to make it through twenty minutes. Whenever she got tired, she floated over to the side of the pool until she caught her breath, then joined the group again.

Frequency: Ronnie started by going to class twice a week, and soon found herself signing up for class five days a week.

To progress her level of fitness, after the first six weeks, Ronnie began alternating riding a stationary bike with her aerobics classes.

Her first *fitness goals* were to make it through an entire forty-five-minute class without taking a time-out, and to improve flexibility in the muscles surrounding her knees.

Her *health goal* was to reduce her knee pain and risk of osteoarthritis by improving her flexibility and losing weight.

To help her stay motivated, Ronnie asked her sister to call her every morning for two weeks to remind her of her commitment to get healthier. She taped the YMCA schedule to her refrigerator as a visual reminder of her new exercise plan.

Need additional motivation to help get out and exercise? Try these tricks:

Take before and after pictures. Before you start your new exercise program, take a photo of yourself in exercise clothes. Take a new "after" picture every few weeks, and notice the improvements in your posture, skin, and muscle tone. Save these in a scrapbook, tape them to your bathroom mirror or refrigerator, or frame them for your bedside table for visual proof of the positive effects of exercise.

Earn credits for time spent exercising. Count your exercise time in "credits" like frequent flier miles. For each hour you exercise, give yourself a point toward whatever "prize" you choose, like a new exercise outfit, a pedicure, or a CD. Better yet, buddy up with a friend, and let her earn credits if you *don't* exercise. There's nothing like knowing you have to buy *her* that handbag you've been coveting to get you off the couch and moving!

WHAT CAN *YOU* EXPECT FROM CARDIOVASCULAR FITNESS?

Both Laurie and Ronnie met their goals, but it took time and perseverance. One of the most common reasons women become discouraged and quit an exercise program is because they don't see the results they expected. Often this is because they never set realistic individual goals. Sometimes even the most sophisticated exerciser can get caught up in the latest celebrity workout plan and expect to wind up looking like the willowy model extolling the latest craze.

Let's face it: only one out of a thousand women are genetically programmed to reach Cindy Crawford's *height*—never mind about her figure! However, it is reasonable for every woman to expect her body to respond positively to an individualized exercise plan. If you follow the program you've created for yourself, you can expect these results at the end of the first four weeks:

What you should see: pink cheeks after exercise, more smiles when you catch your reflection in the mirror, weight loss of a few pounds (don't expect to lose more than one to two pounds a week, even if you are following the nutritional advice in part 4).

What you should feel: slightly looser clothing, anticipation rather than dread when thinking about exercise, a boost in your energy level, more restful sleep.

What you should expect: If you stick with this program, you will decrease your risk of osteoporosis, heart disease, diabetes, high blood pressure, and some cancers.

If you stay at this level of the program and keep it up just thirty minutes five days a week, you will lose an average of ten pounds in the first year if you're overweight at the start. If you are very overweight, you may lose considerably more.

What you should watch out for: If you are exercising with a partner, *pay attention to your exercise intensity.* Be sure you don't inadvertently slow down to a comfortable conversational pace while exercising. One of the advantages of walking with a friend is that you may find time going so quickly that you can increase the *duration* of your exercise sessions. You may decide to go a little slower for a little longer,

FIND AN EXERCISE BUDDY

Need a little extra motivation? Consider finding an exercise buddy. Several studies have shown that women who exercise together are more likely to stick with their exercise program. There can be other benefits, too: Some gyms offer discounted rates for several people joining together, and you can share the cost of other expenses like a baby-sitter. Consider joining a local women's walking group or sports team. If there's not one in your neighborhood, try to get one started.

Don't recruit an exercise partner (including your spouse) who is a lot fitter than you are. Trying to keep up with someone who's always ahead is frustrating and can lead to injury. And if you've been looking for an excuse to get a dog, this is it! There's nothing a pooch likes better than a romp through the neighborhood with his favorite human.

which is fine as long as you stay in your goal THR or RPE zone.

Pay attention to personal safety. If you exercise outside at dusk or dawn, wear white or reflective clothing. Don't let headphones distract you from your surroundings (or from your exercise pace.)

HOW TO FIND THE RIGHT EXERCISE SHOE FOR YOU

When I joined the track team in junior high school, I had to wear a small pair of men's running shoes, because there were no shoes made for female runners. Fast-forward twenty-five years: the only problem now is figuring out which of the many available women's athletic shoes to buy!

Choosing the right exercise shoe may seem like an intimidating process, but it can be easy, and even fun, if you know what to look for.

First, decide what *type* of shoe to buy. If you plan to do one particular type of exercise, buy a shoe designed specifically for that activity, i.e., walking shoes for walkers, running shoes for runners. There really *is* a difference between walking and running shoes. For instance, walking shoes are stiffer and more supportive than running shoes, and usually have a bigger toe box. Running shoes have more cushioning and flexibility, which is crucial for preventing impact-related injuries. If you are thinking about starting with walking and advancing to jogging, go ahead and get a running shoe. But a word of caution: It's okay to walk in running shoes, but you shouldn't run in walking shoes.

There's also a category of shoe called a *cross-trainer,* which has become more popular over the past several years. This is a good shoe for a gym exerciser who might be on the stair machine today, in a stretching class tomorrow, and a step aerobics class the next day. A cross-trainer is a great choice to throw into your suitcase when you're heading off for a vacation or a business trip. A hybrid shoe, it can be used for walking or running a couple of miles occasionally on the treadmill, but is not a good choice for the woman who plans to walk or run frequently. Remember, if you plan to stick primarily with one type of activity, buy a shoe specifically designed for that purpose.

Once you've chosen the type of shoe you need, consider the *shape* of your foot. This is especially important for those buying running shoes. Women tend to have a wider forefoot and narrower heel than men, but just like bodies, feet come in all shapes and sizes. The mold a shoe is built on is called a *last*, which is variably shaped for feet with arches that are flat, high, or normal. Think about the print your foot makes when you walk barefoot on the beach, or when you step out of the shower onto a rug. This can help you decide what the shape of your foot is and guide you in choosing the right shoe. Matching your foot shape to the correct shoe shape can not only make you more comfortable but can help reduce your risk of injury.

Flat arches are the most common type, which are associated with *overpronation,* or excessive rolling inward of the foot. Overpronation can lead to lots of problems with the foot, as well as tendinitis on the inner part of the ankle. Shoes that are built for motion control or stability are best for those with flat feet. On the other end of the spectrum are those with high arches, associated with *supination,* or rolling outward of the foot. Women whose feet supinate benefit from athletic shoes with extra cushioning and a slightly

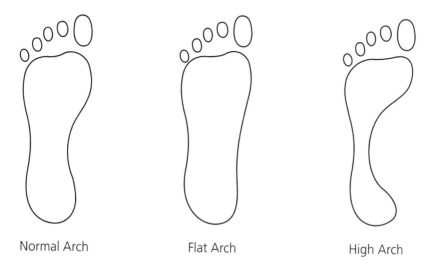

Normal Arch   Flat Arch   High Arch

built-up heel. (Comparison-shop: You'll notice that some athletic shoes have a perfectly flat heel, while others have extra cushioning and height built into the heel.) Those with normal arches can choose from the widest variety of athletic shoes. Be aware that companies that make athletic shoes frequently change shoe design and features. This means that the new version of the shoe you bought last year may be more than just a different color. The Sports Medicine Podiatry Association has a review of currently available models on its Web site. (See References at the back of this book.)

Other Tips for Buying Athletic Shoes

1. *Most women are wearing the wrong size shoes.* When it comes to buying clothing, women have a bad habit of thinking that the smaller the size, the better. Often they assume the same thing with shoes, trying to force their foot into a shoe that's too small. You don't have to be Cinderella to start an exercise program, so leave behind the idea that you need to squeeze into a small shoe size. Go into a reputable athletic shoe store and get your foot measured. Do this at the end of the day when your foot is at its largest, and be sure to wear athletic socks when trying on shoes. And, should you decide to buy a men's shoe, check carefully to be sure the heel is not too wide, or you risk uncomfortable friction blisters.

2. *Don't expect to break in athletic shoes.* Your new shoes will *never feel better* than they do when you try them on in the store. If they don't feel right, don't buy them. With the exception of cleats, you don't have to break in athletic

shoes. Remember, an athletic shoe that feels uncomfortable in the store will *always* feel uncomfortable.

3. *All shoe stores are not created equal.* Most department stores, and even some athletic shoe stores, don't have personnel who really know the difference between one athletic shoe and the next. They can usually measure your foot accurately, so figure out what size you should be shopping for and then look around. There are lots of Internet and mail-order companies, like Athleta and Road Runner Sports, that are happy to share their expert knowledge of their products.

4. *Never, never, never* exercise in shoes that aren't intended for athletic activity. This includes our beloved Keds, which are fine for a stroll in the park but aren't built for anything more challenging.

5. *Go shopping.* Get new shoes frequently. One of the most common contributing factors to many of the injuries I see is a worn-out shoe. Athletic shoes are tough; they're built to withstand a lot of pounding, jumping, and sliding. But don't wait until there are holes in the tread before replacing them! Running or walking shoes should be replaced every 350 to 500 miles, or once a year, whichever comes first. For a sport like tennis, how often you get new shoes depends on how often you play. Replace your shoes once a year if you play once a week, twice a year if you play twice a week, and so on. The midsole of any athletic shoe (between the footbed and outer sole) has only so much cushioning power in it before it starts to fail, leaving you more vulnerable to injury. It's also vulnerable to the passage of time and environmental influences, especially temperature fluctuations. So don't bother dusting off those old unworn shoes

sitting on the top shelf of your closet. Treat yourself to a new pair of athletic shoes.

6. *Buy a shoe, not an advertisement.* Some companies put tons of money behind the marquee stars who advertise their products. But just because one shoe is right for a recognizable face doesn't mean it's right for your foot. Case in point: Nike, whose running shoes tend to be too narrow in the toe box for many female runners. Comparison-shop, and try shoes like Saucony, whose roomy toe boxes are a terrific fit for the average female foot, or New Balance, which offers a choice of widths.

THE FASHION FACTOR

The good news: There are no fashion police looking over your shoulder while you exercise. Gone are the matching leotards and leg warmers that marked the aerobics craze in the past two decades. Today's emphasis in fitness wear is on comfort and performance. All you need is a good pair of athletic shoes and comfortable clothing (whether loose or form-fitted is up to you). But rather than cotton, which stays stuck to your skin with sweat, try exercise clothing made of fabric treated to wick moisture away from your body. Some brands to look for include CoolMax or Power Dry polyester and Supplex nylon. And for those who remember the *Rocky* movies, remember this: Wearing heavy sweats will *not* help you to lose weight faster. They will only make you sweat a lot, resulting in dehydration, and leaving you feeling tired or light-headed—all of which will conspire to cut your workout short.

HOW TO EAT FOR EXERCISE

Unless you're going to exercise for a prolonged period (more than sixty minutes), you don't need to eat before you exercise, as long as you haven't gone more than a few hours without food. If it has been several hours since your last meal or snack, or you exercise first thing in the morning, it's a good idea to fuel up. After several hours, your blood sugar dips, and your workout may be hampered by fatigue, nausea, or poor performance (and in that case, why bother exercising?).

If you're going to have a snack before exercise, go for a snack that's 150 to 350 calories. A mix of protein and carbohydrate is usually a good way to go, like turkey on half a bagel, fruit with yogurt, or fig bars and skim milk. Some people are able to tolerate more fat than others before exercise, which makes trail mix or peanut butter crackers options to

---

What about energy bars?
Energy bars, or sports bars as they are sometimes known, first became popular in the 1980s with the development of Power-Bar. Now there are at least twenty different brands in flavors from berry to brownie. They provide anywhere from 100 to over 300 calories, many of which are from sugar. Despite their popularity, they don't provide energy that's superior to the energy you'd get from a banana, fig bars, or other food, *and* they miss out on many of the nutrients you get from food. Bottom line? Any energy source is better than no energy source, but don't use these bars in place of meals.

---

consider. Don't be afraid to experiment and see what works for you.

If you don't want to eat solid food, try a sports drink. The glucose will speed into your bloodstream, providing almost instant energy. For a homemade version of a sports drink, mix an ounce or two of juice (consider trying cranberry, grape, or pineapple) with half a cup of water.

CHAPTER 4

LIFE'S TWISTS AND TURNS: MAINTAINING FLEXIBILITY

Andrea is a thirty-eight-year-old accountant who began to notice some stiffness in her back during the last tax season. She thought it was just a result of sitting long hours, but even after her schedule lightened up she continued to have pain. She came in for a checkup, worried that she was developing a more serious problem, like arthritis.

IF YOU'RE LIKE ANDREA (and a lot of my patients are), there's a good chance that even before you begin your new exercise program, you may be complaining of feeling stiff. Countless young women have asked me to evaluate them for arthritis because they wake up each morning feeling like an "old lady," grumbling about being stiff and achy. These women don't have arthritis, but they are the poster gals for that old saying "If you don't move it, you lose it" . . . flexibility, that is. To understand how this happens, we need to take a look at the human skeleton.

YOUR BODY'S "SCAFFOLDING"

The skeleton is made up of 206 bones that are fastened together by thick bands of connective tissue called *ligaments*. The skeleton is a rigid framework that protects the internal organs like the heart, lungs, and brain, but at the same time it is a wonderfully flexible structure that allows movement. Movement occurs only at the intersection of two or more bones in a *joint*. Our joints are lined with a lubricated smooth surface called *cartilage*. Muscles attach to bones by thick bands of fibrous tissue called *tendons*, and provide the power for joints to glide through a normal range of motion. Every movement—from walking to picking up a child to throwing a ball—relies on this range of motion.

Each muscle is surrounded by a tough layer of fibrous connective tissue called *fascia*. Stretching increases the flexibility of this connective tissue, as well as elongating the muscle and its tendon (remember, the tendon is the "rope" that attaches the muscle to bone). The primary effect of stretching is on the fascia and tendon, which become more *elastic*. Keeping muscles and tendons flexible helps maintain your joints' ability to move freely. When muscles aren't stretched, they become less flexible, which leads to limitations in the joints' range of motion. That limitation is what causes patients to complain of feeling stiff. This is precisely what had happened to my patient, Andrea. She had a sedentary job and didn't exercise. Over the years, her muscles became less flexible, and she lost the free range of motion of her joints. A simple stretching program restored her muscle flexibility and joint range of motion, and worked like a charm to get rid of her pain.

THE HEALTH AND FITNESS
BENEFITS OF STRETCHING

Stretching can certainly make you move more comfortably, and many athletes firmly believe that regular stretching improves athletic performance. However, although most sports medicine doctors recommend stretching as a part of a total fitness program, whether or not stretching actually prevents athletic injuries is a topic of controversy. Multiple studies have not shown that flexibility decreases injury rates (although many of these studies have not included female athletes). Many athletes, including the U.S. Women's National Soccer Team, stretch after every workout session, and some believe this practice has helped keep their injury rates down. My personal experience has been that athletic injuries are often seen in those who either have imbalances in flexibility (for instance, the quadriceps muscle in the front of the thigh is fairly flexible, but the hamstrings and calf muscles in the back of the leg are not) or have generally poor flexibility overall. Whether or not this is actually a cause of injury or just an association isn't clear.

What is not controversial is that stretching provides many benefits and is an important ingredient to incorporate into your new fitness program. Stretching clearly helps maintain joint range of motion, which is especially important as we age. I can't count the times a patient has complained of stiffness, followed by an offhand remark like "I guess I'm just getting old." But it has nothing to do with getting old and everything to do with lost flexibility.

Recent studies have shown that stretching can improve athletic performance, and others have shown that stretching after weight lifting helps make you stronger than weight lifting alone can. One study even showed that stretching alone—without ever lifting a weight—could improve strength. Stretching helps to decrease the muscle tightness associated with exercise and has been shown to be an effective stress reliever. Stretching is also a mainstay of sports physical therapists' treatment for injuries.

HOW ARTHRITIS BENEFITS FROM FLEXIBILITY EXERCISES

There are several types of arthritis, many of which have causes rooted in the immune system. *Osteoarthritis* is a different type of arthritis, not associated with the immune system but rather with *mechanical* breakdown in the cartilage that normally cushions joints. Also called degenerative joint disease, osteoarthritis is by far the most common type of arthritis and is particularly prevalent among women.

Osteoarthritis may be caused by an injury to a joint, and as such is sometimes called *traumatic arthritis*. However, osteoarthritis is most commonly associated with excess weight. This is because too much weight on the skeletal system puts excess pressure on the joints, causing them to collapse or become too narrow. As the joint collapses, the lubricating and cushioning cartilage is slowly crushed, and the joint loses its normal range of motion.

Gentle stretching of the muscles around an arthritic joint can help to offset this, preserving the joint's range of motion. Flexibility exercises have also been found to be an effective form of pain relief for many women with mild to moderate arthritis.

DESIGNING YOUR OWN
FLEXIBILITY FITNESS PLAN

One of the questions I ask patients is "How much do you stretch?" The answer I hear most frequently is "Not as much as I should." Many of them have the perception that stretching is like flossing one's teeth: a good thing to do, but not much fun. But once someone's suffered the consequences of lost flexibility (or lost teeth), she's sure to wish she had practiced a little preventive medicine. So use the tests below to evaluate your own flexibility. Then plan to maintain the range of motion you have by stretching two or three days a week, or choose to stretch more frequently to improve your elasticity.

Evaluating Your Flexibility

1. Wearing loose-fitting, comfortable clothing, sit on the floor with your legs out in front of you, feet about a foot apart. Place a measuring tape, yardstick, or ruler on the floor between your feet so that it is parallel to your legs (see illustration on page 86). Line the one-inch mark up with your ankles. Lean forward, stretching out your arms and hands in front of you. See if you can reach past your ankles. Touch the measuring stick and write down the highest number you can reach. This gives you a general idea of your overall flexibility, but specifically of the muscles of your back and the muscles in the back of your thighs and calves. If you weren't able to reach your ankles at all, or could just barely touch them, you should consider doing stretches for the back and legs several days a week. Then do this flexibility test again in four weeks to see how you measure up. If you could reach several inches (five or more) past your ankles, your overall flexibility is

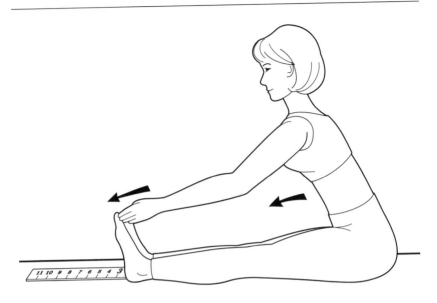

better than the average woman. You should perform the stretches at least three days a week to maintain your flexibility, or stretch more frequently if you'd like to improve it.

2. Stand straight, with your arms dangling by your sides and a *slight* bend in your knees. Lean to your left, dropping your hand down the side of your leg. (Be sure your right foot doesn't come off the floor). See how close your fingertips come to your knees (see opposite). Now straighten back up and lean toward your right. Again, this gives you an idea of your general flexibility, specifically of your back and the sides of your hips and legs. If your fingertips don't come close to reaching your knees, you need to spend extra time working on your flexibility.

3. Stand with your left hand holding on to a door frame for support (see illustration on page 88). Tighten the muscles in your abdomen (stomach) and buttocks. Bend your right knee behind you, and grasp your right ankle with your

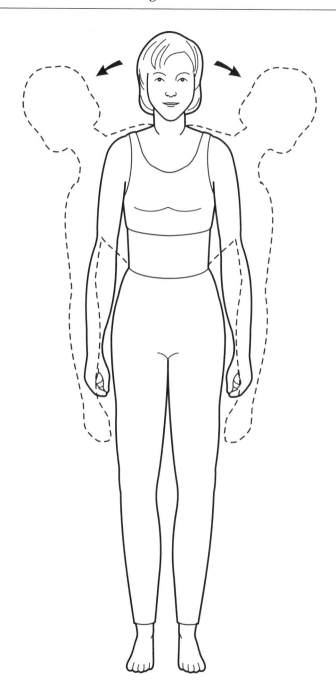

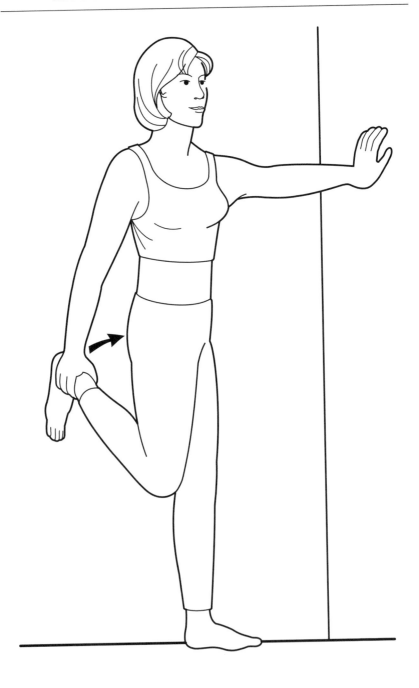

right hand. Keeping your right knee in line with your right hip, gently pull your heel toward your buttock. Your goal should be to touch your heel to your buttock. If you can't, you should spend extra time working on your quadriceps, the big muscle group in the front of the thigh.

LET'S GET STRETCHING!

To get started on a flexibility program, let's apply the same five fitness factors we used for cardiovascular fitness.

1. Type of Activity

What type of stretches you should do is probably the most hotly debated question in regard to stretching. Stretches generally fall into one of three categories: *static, ballistic,* and *proprioceptive neuromuscular facilitation* (PNF, for short).

Static stretches are the classical style of stretching that most people are familiar with and involve slowly stretching the muscle and tendon, holding the stretch for several seconds, and then relaxing. Ballistic, or "bouncing," stretches involve stretching and relaxing the muscle and tendon quickly and repetitively, and have generally fallen out of favor because of the concern that they may precipitate injury. The last category, PNF, is a combination of muscle contraction (held for six seconds) followed by passive stretching (for at least ten seconds). The latter is probably the most effective but also the most complicated. It requires a partner and more practice to master. For the average woman, static stretches like the ones illustrated in this chapter are the best bet.

2. Intensity

Sometimes a patient will complain to me that she "can't feel" a stretch. This means either that the particular muscle she's stretching is already quite flexible or that she's doing the stretch incorrectly. A beginner will almost always feel the stretch. To stretch a muscle with appropriate intensity, begin your stretch and hold it when you reach a point of resistance (you should feel tension but not pain). If it feels uncomfortable, relax the stretch a bit. After a few seconds, you may feel the muscle loosen up slightly, at which point you may want to try to gently stretch it a little farther. STRETCHES SHOULD NEVER BE PAINFUL. If a stretch is causing you pain, ask your doctor, a physical therapist, or some other exercise professional to check your form.

Should I stretch before or after exercise?

Don't confuse stretching with warming up and cooling down! Because exercise raises your body temperature, muscles become "warmer" and more pliable with exercise. Traditionally, it's thought that muscles are most receptive to stretching—and least likely to be injured—when they are in this "warmed" state. But studies have not confirmed that *when* you stretch really makes a significant difference in overall flexibility. Despite the lack of scientific agreement, stretching after exercise, when the muscles are warm from increased blood flow, seems logical to me. Many people feel they "get a better stretch" if the muscles are warm, but I have plenty of patients who start their day with a short stretching routine as soon as they roll out of bed. Try both ways and see what works for you.

---

3. Duration

Begin by holding each stretch for ten seconds, then relax and repeat. Work up to holding a stretch for thirty seconds. I usually recommend three or four repetitions of each stretch. Nobody knows how many repetitions are optimal, but at least one good study found range of motion didn't improve much after four repetitions. It won't take much of your time to stretch effectively: you can stretch each muscle for just one or two minutes two or three times a week (see below) to improve your joint range of motion.

4. Frequency

Unlike cardiovascular exercise, the recommendations for stretching are not very specific. This is partly due to the difficulty we've had with deciding exactly what "normal" flexibility is. When compared to men, women tend to have more joint laxity (sometimes known as being loose-jointed), which can be difficult to separate from flexibility of the muscle and tendon. The American College of Sports Medicine recommends stretching the major muscle groups, such as the quadriceps, hamstrings, and calves, "enough to maintain range of motion," two to three days a week.

How often you personally decide to stretch depends on the degree of flexibility you already have, and what your chosen activity is. For instance, dancing generally requires more flexibility than riding a bicycle, so if dancing is your primary form of exercise, you may choose to spend more time working on flexibility. Similarly, if you plan to start a walking program, you may want to focus primarily on stretching the back and legs and very little time on your upper body. Many women benefit from performing flexibility exercises daily.

5. Progression

Initially, build on your flexibility program by increasing the duration of each stretch, from ten seconds to thirty or more seconds. Then do so by adding new stretches, varying your routine. Consider taking a class that emphasizes stretching, like a stretching-and-toning class or yoga. Experiment with devices like stretching cords, slant boards, and fitness balls, all designed to add variety to your fitness program.

YOGA

Say the word *yoga*, and many people conjure up an image of a woman dressed in white, sitting cross-legged on a mat, eyes closed in meditation. But yoga enthusiasts know that there are literally dozens of styles of yoga, ranging from the serene, calm-and-flexibility-inducing type to a vigorous, aerobic muscle-pumping type of workout. Whichever style catches your attention, yoga can be used to increase flexibility, reduce anxiety, improve posture, tone muscles, and lower blood pressure. It has even been used to help people quit smoking! Interested? Check your local telephone directory for a yoga studio near you, contact the experts at Collage Video for a comparison of current videotapes, or log on to www.yogasite.com.

WRITE IT DOWN

Again, keeping the five fitness factors in mind, complete the worksheet below. This will be Part Two of your personal exercise program. You can use the sample stretches illustrated in the following pages for guidance. In addition to improving your general flexibility, be sure to pay special attention to any muscles you find are particularly tight. For instance, if you wear high heels frequently, you are likely to have especially tight muscles in your calves, and you should stretch them more frequently. If you do a lot of desk work, chances are you need to do more flexibility exercises for your low back and hamstrings (muscles in the back of the thigh).

Part Two of My Personal Exercise Program

Flexibility Exercises

Results of my first flexibility assessment:

Which muscles or stretches I'm going to focus on:

When I'm going to do them:

My flexibility goals include:

My health goals include:

To help stay motivated, I will:

SAMPLE STRETCHING EXERCISES

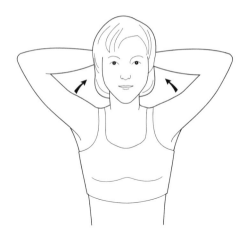

Shoulders/Front of Arms

1. Place your hands on the back of your head, palms facing forward.
2. Press your arms back until you feel a stretch in your chest and shoulders.
3. Hold 10 seconds. Repeat 2 to 3 times.

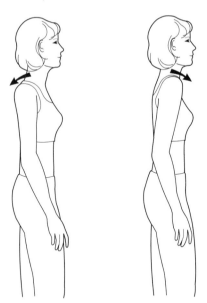

Shoulders

1. Stand straight with shoulders relaxed.
2. Slowly roll shoulders backward.
3. Pause, then slowly roll shoulders forward.
4. Repeat 2 to 3 times.

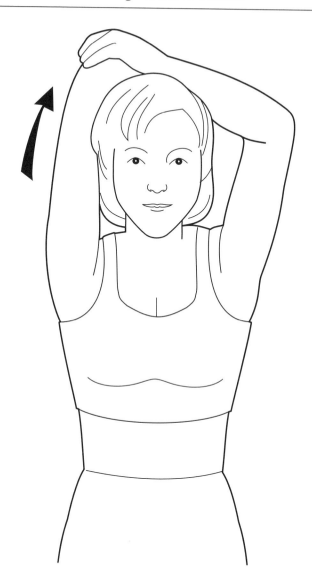

Triceps

1. Hold your right elbow with your left hand, as shown.
2. Pull the elbow behind your head until you feel a stretch in the back of the right arm.
3. Hold 10 seconds.
4. Switch arms.
5. Repeat 2 to 3 times with each arm.

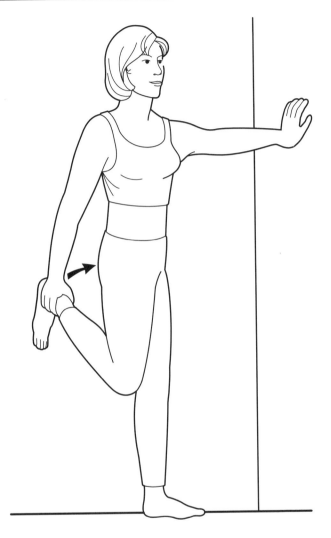

Quadriceps

1. Hold your right ankle, as shown.
2. Keep knees parallel and tuck your buttocks under.
3. Gently pull your right ankle toward your buttocks.
4. Do not lean forward or allow the back to arch.
5. Hold 10 to 30 seconds.
6. Switch legs.
7. Repeat 2 to 3 times for each leg.

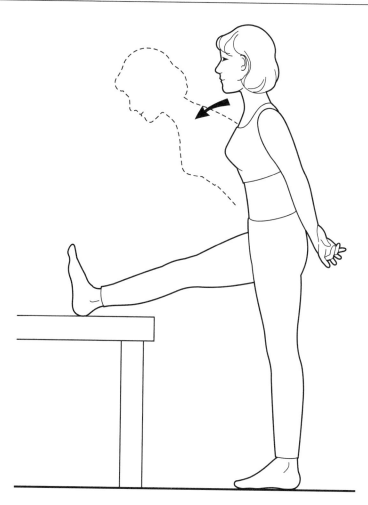

Hamstrings

1. Place your right leg on a table or bench at a height comfortable for you. Keep your knee straight and your toes pointed up.
2. Stand straight with your buttocks and hips tucked under.
3. Bend forward at your hip, keeping your back straight.
4. Feel the stretch in the back of your right thigh. (You will also feel some stretch in the calf.)
5. Hold 10 to 30 seconds.
6. Switch legs.
7. Repeat 2 to 3 times with each leg.

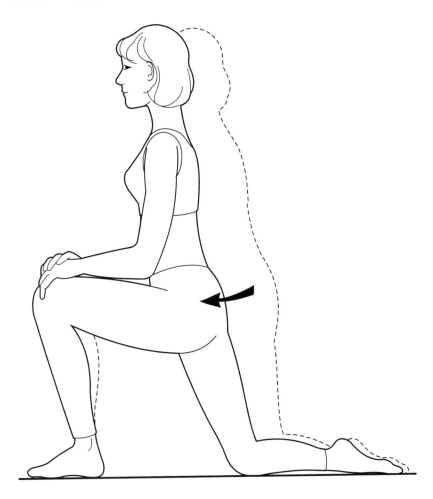

Hips

1. Take a big step forward with your left leg. Lower your body to the floor, as shown.
2. Keep your chest upright. Shift your torso forward. Be sure to keep your left knee behind your toes.
3. Feel a stretch in the front of the right hip.
4. Hold 10 to 30 seconds.
5. Switch sides.
6. Repeat 2 to 3 times with each leg.

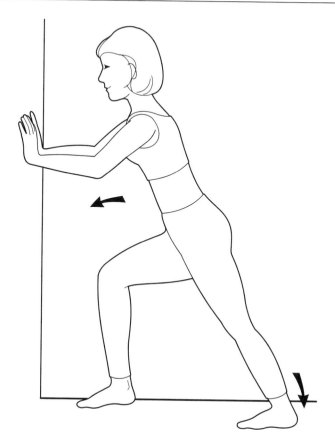

Calves

1. Place your hands against a wall, and position your body as shown, keeping your toes pointed straight ahead.
2. Keep your left (back) heel down.
3. Lean into the wall, keeping your left knee straight until you feel a stretch in your calf.
4. Hold 10 to 30 seconds.
5. Switch sides.
6. Repeat 2 to 3 times with each leg.

Note: If you bend the back knee, keeping the heel on the ground, you'll get a really good stretch of the calf and Achilles tendon (the back of the heel). This is an especially good stretch for women who wear high heels.

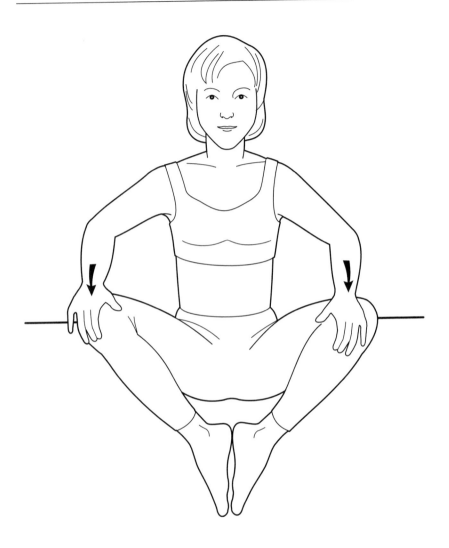

Groin

1. Sit up straight with your feet together, as shown.
2. Use your hands to gently press your knees downward toward the floor until you feel a stretch in your inner thighs and groin.
3. Hold 10 to 30 seconds. Repeat 2 to 3 times.

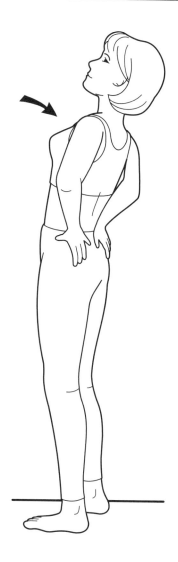

Lower Back

1. Place your hands against your lower back, fingers pointing down, as shown.
2. Bend backward gently until you feel a stretch in your lower back.
3. Hold 10 seconds. Repeat 2 to 3 times.
4. You can do this exercise several times daily, particularly after prolonged sitting or forward bending.

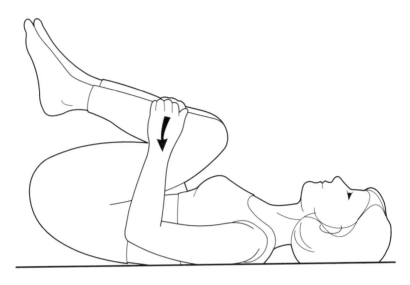

Alternate Lower Back Stretch

1. Lie on your back with your head and shoulders relaxed on the floor.
2. Gently pull both knees to your chest.
3. Hold 10 to 30 seconds. Repeat 2 to 3 times.

WHAT CAN *YOU* EXPECT FROM FLEXIBILITY EXERCISES?

Many women have told me that, despite their good intentions, they find themselves skipping the stretching part of their exercise programs. Most of them say this is because they are pressed for time and want to spend every minute they have available for exercise on calorie-burning cardiovascular exercise. But even the busiest woman has a few minutes during the day into which she can slip a few stretches, because stretching exercises are the ultimate "multitasking" type of exercise. Be creative! Stretch when you're talking on the phone, watching television, or waiting for food to cook.

Keep your commitment to this important part of your fitness program and in just a few weeks you'll see the following results:

What you should see: A more relaxed you! You also may see an improvement in posture.

What you should feel: Stress relief, less muscle tightness and overall stiffness, joints that move more comfortably. You may also notice an improvement in athletic performance and strength.

What you should expect: If you stick with stretching exercises, especially as you age, you can expect less joint pain and muscle stiffness, even if you suffer from arthritis. You will also have reduced your chance of developing low back pain.

What you should watch out for: Stay away from stretches that are ballistic (i.e., don't bounce), as these increase the risk of injury. Remember, stretching should never be painful.

CHAPTER 5

HEALTHY MUSCLES, BONES, AND METABOLISM: THE POWER OF STRENGTH TRAINING

"I DON'T WANT TO get bigger and bulkier!"

"I'm too old to try weight training."

"Lifting weights is for real athletes."

More often than not, I hear one of these dismissive comments from women when I bring up the topic of strength training. Sadly, their attitudes are based on myths. The truth is that strength training, also called *resistance* or *weight training*, is beneficial for *every woman*, no matter what her age or fitness level is. And rather than causing women to get bigger, weight training generally leads to a smaller, "tighter" physique.

More important, weight training is an almost magical way to achieve many of your health goals. Recent research has shown that weight training can be good for the cardiovascular system, can improve or prevent osteoporosis, can reduce the chance of developing diabetes, and can elevate mood. It also appears to improve our balance, reducing the risk of bone-breaking falls as we age. But for many women, the most attractive aspect of weight training is that it is a very effective way to lose weight and maintain a trimmer body.

MUSCLES ARE RESPONSIBLE FOR MOVEMENT AND METABOLISM

There are over 600 muscles in the human body, ranging in size from mere fractions of an inch to a few feet in length. Approximately one-third of the average woman's body weight comes from these muscles, which are largely made up of protein and water. The muscle tissue forms in strands we call fibers and are smaller in women than in men. There are two types of these fibers: *slow twitch* and *fast twitch*. Generally, slow twitch fibers are used for most of our activities, although fast twitch fibers often initiate movement and are called into play when we increase the intensity of activity. Slow twitch fibers are dependent on oxygen for energy. Fast twitch fibers can work without oxygen, but not for long.

When you use a muscle for average daily activity, like strolling across the street or putting groceries away, blood flow to the working muscles increases, bringing in the oxygen needed for energy. But when you use the muscle more forcefully—to race across the street, for instance—the sudden powerful contraction of the muscles essentially blocks blood flowing in. This is why you need those fast twitch fibers that can work in the absence of oxygen (*anaerobically*).

As we age, we lose some of our muscle mass. Many studies have concluded that *this occurs primarily because fast twitch fibers shrink in size.* This process usually begins to occur in our thirties or forties, and continues each year thereafter. In my interactions with patients, I frequently hear them joke about their "muscle turning into fat." In reality, what's happening is that muscle shrinks, and fat takes its place, filling in the space where the muscle used to be.

This has two consequences. The first is that as those muscle fibers shrink, you lose power. You move more slowly and begin to have trouble lifting anything heavy. Eventually, you lose so many fast twitch fibers that you have difficulty doing anything, which accounts for those elderly relatives who have difficulty even getting up from a chair. This leads to loss of independence, and is unfortunately the main reason many women end up in nursing homes. The second consequence of this loss of muscle tissue is that our metabolism slows down, leading to weight (fat) gain. To do their jobs efficiently, muscles require a lot of energy, which is provided by the foods we eat. But once we've lost that muscle tissue, we don't need as much food anymore, so more of the food we eat gets stored as fat.

But *loss of muscle is not an inevitable part of aging,* as we once thought. Use your muscles, especially the fast twitch ones, and you can largely prevent this sad state of affairs from ever occurring! And even if you're past fifty, and your muscle fibers have already become shrunken, you can reverse that process by strength training. No matter what your age or level of physical functioning, weight training can be safe and effective.

HOW STRENGTH TRAINING
AFFECTS BONE HEALTH

Not only does strength training build strong muscles, it helps build strong bones as well. While bones may look solid to the naked eye, under the microscope they appear full of small holes, or *pores,* much like a sponge or a piece of Swiss cheese. The number of pores in the bone can be affected by a wide variety of factors, including age, heredity, diet, hormones, medications, and activity level. Too many pores means the bone has a decreased *density,* leaving it fragile, brittle, and easily broken. This condition is known as *osteoporosis* (*osteo* means bone, *porosis* refers to the pores) and affects several million American women.

The groundbreaking research done by Miriam Nelson, Ph.D., author of *Strong Women Stay Young,* and her colleagues at Tufts University showed us that weight training is one of the best soldiers we have in the fight against osteoporosis. Their research confirmed that strength training can stimulate the bone to both prevent and reverse the loss of bone seen in osteoporosis. At the time of this writing, we really don't know exactly how strength training does this. Weight training increases amounts of various hormones in the bloodstream, several of which probably have a positive effect on the bone's density. Additionally, when you lift a weight, the muscle's tendon pulls on its attachment to bone, which seems to encourage bone cells to proliferate.

It appears that weight-bearing exercises like walking stimulate bone through physical impact. However, studies show that walking is associated with an increased bone mass at the hip, but *not* at the spine, which is the single most important measurement doctors use to predict risk of fractures. Weight training, however, seems to promote increased bone density throughout the skeleton, decreasing such risk.

Although the landmark Surgeon General's first report of physical activity and health states that it is too soon to draw conclusions from the early studies of weight training and osteoporosis, I personally recommend strength training for all women, including those with or at risk for osteoporosis. But be patient: It takes several months of consistent strengthening to be able to detect any change. Yet again, a reminder of why it's important that you design an exercise program you can stick with.

RISK FACTORS FOR OSTEOPOROSIS

Female gender
Caucasian or Asian ethnicity
Age (the older you get, the greater your risk)
Small frame: weight less than 127 pounds
Eating disorder, whether past or present
Family history of the disease
Inadequate dietary calcium and vitamin D
Early menopause (before age forty-five)
Sedentary lifestyle
Smoking
Two or more drinks of alcohol daily

TAI CHI

Did you know that our sense of balance starts to fall off when we're in our forties? For a woman with osteoporosis, this is more than just an annoyance, because losing balance means an increased risk of bone-breaking falls.

Enter tai chi, a type of exercise that has become increasingly popular in the last few years, especially among women with osteoporosis and their doctors. Tai chi is an ancient Chinese practice that combines physical activity, controlled breathing, and mental concentration. Not only has tai chi been found to improve balance, it also has been reported to improve cardiorespiratory function, decrease arthritis pain, and reduce depression.

ADDITIONAL HEALTH BENEFITS OF STRENGTH TRAINING

When I ask patients about their goals for strength training, the first response I get is often a blank look. But when they glimpse the realm of possibilities afforded by strength training, they quickly become animated. Some women simply wish to preserve their functional independence—to be able to walk four blocks home from the store carrying two bags of groceries; others want to develop the muscular stamina to enjoy a weeklong biking, hiking, or kayaking trip. One of my patients "just wanted enough energy to get through the day," but ended up so pleased with the results of weight training that she joined a group of women training for an amateur body-building competition.

Any woman who strength trains can expect to end up stronger and more energetic and with more muscle tone and definition: a firmer fanny, less flabby arms, sleeker legs. But that's just the "window dressing," because the main benefits of strength training are related to improved health. In addition to building stronger bones, weight training boosts your health in a variety of other ways:

- Recent studies show us that strength training *alone* can lower blood pressure by an average of 2 to 4 percent; a combination of cardiovascular exercise and strength training is even more effective.
- Researchers have found that strength training decreases anger, anxiety, and depression, probably through a positive effect on the mood-stimulating chemicals in the brain.
- Even sufferers of arthritis seem to benefit from strength training. Studies reveal that those with arthritis report less pain when placed on a strength-training program. This seems to be due to improved joint range of motion, although it may also be related to strength training's positive effect on mood.

BREAKING THE BARRIERS TO STRENGTH TRAINING

Women often have a tendency to read a book like this one and immediately start to say "I can't," especially when it comes to a new idea like weight training. But you *can*. My professional experience is that women who have never weight trained have one common barrier they must overcome: the intimidation factor. If you are still hesitating, even after reading about all the wonderful things strength training can do for you, think hard about *why*. Be honest with yourself. Contrary to many women's fears, you don't need any previous exercise experience. And you will get tremendous health benefits from weight training without spending much at all in time or money.

Women are wonderfully resourceful when it comes to problem solving for other members of the family; they just need to take the time to find solutions to their own obstacles. Be creative! The following examples may help you to deal with your concerns.

FACT VS. FICTION: THE TRUTH ABOUT STRENGTH TRAINING

Louise is a forty-two-year-old nurse with mild high blood pressure. At 5'7'' and 170 pounds, she wanted to exercise for weight loss and blood pressure control. She had begun a walking program and wanted advice about alternate exercises to meet her goals. She was dumbfounded when I suggested strength training.

"Oh yeah, right, me and the Incredible Hulk exercising together!"

That was Louise's response when I suggested she add weight training to her walking program. She was initially skeptical, and very concerned that weight lifting would just make her look bigger. But the irony is that Louise, like most women, couldn't develop big muscles just by lifting weights even if she tried. Men naturally have much larger muscles primarily because of the male hormone, testosterone, which stimulates muscles to grow in size. All women have a small amount of testosterone, and some have more than others. But even a woman who has much more testosterone than the average still has just a tiny fraction of the amount a man has, and won't end up with big bulky muscles.

The Truth About Female Bodybuilders

When I tried to reassure Louise that she wouldn't bulk up, she asked, "Well then, what about those female bodybuilders I've seen?" She was referring to a small group of women who are abusing their bodies by taking steroids, growth hormone, and other unsafe substances, with the express purpose of building unnaturally large muscles. A few of my patients are professional competitive bodybuilders, and their visits to my office tell the story. They have abnormal growth of facial and chest hair, deepening voices, and develop dangerous liver, kidney, and heart problems. These are side effects of steroids, and tragically they may not be reversible even if the woman stops using these destructive medications.

There are "natural" bodybuilders as well, women who shun drug use but have unusually well-developed muscles. For these women to achieve such big muscles, they must have a genetic predisposition for developing larger muscles than the average woman, and must work out with *very heavy weights* for several hours each week. And remember, the appearance of a bodybuilder striking a pose during a bodybuilding competition can be deceiving. A competitive bodybuilder spends hours developing muscle control so she can create an illusion of power simply by "rippling" a muscle. She may profoundly limit her dietary intake for weeks before the competition, which results in fat loss and makes the muscles stand out even more. Some bodybuilders purposefully dehydrate themselves so that skin appears thin and tight over their muscles. This is what's caught on film and creates your impression of a bodybuilder. But if you saw the same woman a few weeks later, after she's eating and drinking normally again, her muscles would appear much less defined.

Trust me. You can't develop muscles like a bodybuilder without trying very, very hard.

FOR WEIGHT LOSS, CARDIOVASCULAR EXERCISE ISN'T ENOUGH

Karen, a thirty-five-year-old attorney, began taking aerobic dance classes to combat job-related stress and to help control her weight. She started her program two years ago, beginning with an easy class once a week, and gradually progressed until she was going three days a week to an advanced class. She tried dieting as well, but despite "doing everything right," she was frustrated by her inability to lose weight.

Karen was initially very resistant to the idea of weight training. She thought that aerobic dance should give her plenty of muscle strength, but she was wrong. Her aerobic exercise was great for her heart, and it probably contributed to improving her muscle endurance, but she needed to add strength training exercises to really stimulate her muscles and boost her metabolism for weight loss.

How does this work? There are two ways that strength training can impact weight loss. The first and most direct is the impact on the muscle itself. Like our bones, skin, and other organs, muscle tissue is constantly in the process of change. It mends any area of injured tissue through a complicated system of repair, laying down new layers of muscle fibers in place of worn or injured ones. Strength training stresses muscle, which stimulates this repair mechanism.

Muscles are very *metabolically active,* meaning that they use up a lot of calories. They burn calories not just while you're exercising, but even when you're resting. So building more calorie-burning muscle through strength training means that you'll boost the number of calories you use throughout the day—you'll even burn extra calories when you're sleeping! This is in stark contrast to fat, which I liken to a parasite: it hangs around you, requiring you furnish it with a blood supply for the delivery of oxygen and other nutrients, and it doesn't do much to support itself. But the worst part is that by increasing your risk of cardiovascular disease, diabetes, and other diseases, your fat is slowly killing you.

Ironically, Karen's dieting was one of the reasons she couldn't lose weight. When she dieted, she lost some fat *but also lost muscle.* And that loss of muscle meant the number of calories she burned in a day actually *went down.* Strength training was the best way for her to regain calorie-burning muscle.

A Pound of Marshmallows vs. a Pound of Lead

As muscles develop, they demand more energy. Your body gradually uses extra fat stores to supply your muscles with the fuel they need. This results in *fat loss,* but not necessarily in *weight loss.* Women who strength train end up losing inches rather than weight. *It's very important to realize* that as you strength train, your weight on the scale may not change much, or may even increase, because you are essentially making a "trade" of fat for muscle. Karen had to remember this as she began strength training. She had to learn to rely on the fact that her clothes were getting looser rather than following numbers on a scale. I told her to think of a pound of muscle like a pound of lead, compact and solid, whereas a pound of fat takes up a lot of space, like a pound of marshmallows. She readily agreed that she'd rather have a firm, solid body rather than look like a giant marshmallow. So remember, if you add a pound of muscle and lose a pound of fat, the number on the scale won't change. But your calorie needs will increase, you will eventually lose a few pounds of fat, and you'll find you're able to eat more without gaining an ounce!

The other way that strength training can impact weight loss is more indirect, but it's also very important. As you get stronger, it's easier to perform your cardiovascular activities. This allows you to increase your intensity level or the duration of exercise, both of which allow you to burn additional calories. And as you age, continued strength training boosts your energy, allowing you to remain active. In the long run, it may be this last benefit that is most essential to good health.

YOU'RE NEVER TOO OLD TO
TRY STRENGTH TRAINING

Margaret is a sixty-four-year-old woman whose mother suffered from osteoporosis. Margaret worked diligently on decreasing her risk of the same disease by paying careful attention to her diet, walking several days weekly, and stopping smoking. When her recent bone density test showed early osteoporosis, she came in to ask if she should change her exercise program.

Margaret was flabbergasted when I suggested weight training. She echoed a concern that I hear commonly from women over forty: "I'm too old to lift weights!" Many of the current baby boomers went to high school at a time when cheerleading was often the only acceptable form of physical activity for women. Today, most women of this generation feel good about the advances of women in sports, and many do some form of cardiovascular exercise, like walking. But weight lifting, they tell me, seems like an activity for the young and strong.

Research in the past couple of decades indicates that this belief couldn't be more wrong. Somewhere after our thirtieth birthday we begin to lose muscle, and unless we reverse this downward slide, we'll end up losing about half a pound or more every year. Looking at tests like CAT scans and MRIs of women who typify this pattern is depressing: I see plenty of fluffy fat filling in where muscle used to be; the muscle appears thin, small, and neglected. The good news, however, is that this pattern is surprisingly easy to reverse.

The most significant factor in loss of muscle size and strength with aging is *lack of use.* Several researchers have found that women who weight train easily increase their muscle tissue, ending up leaner, stronger, and healthier than women many years younger. And these improvements can been seen in *just a few weeks.* Most researchers note significant change within eight to twelve weeks. One study even reported a doubling of strength in just four weeks!

When I asked Margaret why her age was a concern, I expected her to say that she was afraid of getting hurt. But what she said was simply that she thought she'd be embarrassed to be seen in a weight room. She was very happy to know that strength training could be done at home, with very inexpensive equipment. For women who are concerned about getting injured, the findings of Tufts University researcher Dr. Miriam Nelson are very reassuring. Dr. Nelson evaluated weight training's effects on many older women, some of whom were well into their eighties. Those women noticed a lot of changes—improvements in their energy, balance, and strength, for starters—but not one of them reported an injury. My personal experience has been similar: About half of my patients weight train, but I see very few related injuries. When I do see such an injury, it usually is simply a result of overenthusiasm and resolves with a few days of rest.

DESIGNING YOUR STRENGTH-TRAINING PROGRAM

Although weight training is a subject of great interest and has been the topic of thousands of magazine articles, books, and lectures, it has also generated lots of debate. I have listened to well-respected clinicians argue about "normal" strength. For the woman who is simply trying to improve her own health, deciding what's normal for the general population doesn't really make much sense. All that matters is that you know what your starting point is so that you can measure your own progress.

To get an idea of the current shape of your muscles, try the following simple exercises. Again, this is a test that you can do at home, with a friend or by yourself. Write down the results of your first muscle-strength and endurance tests on the worksheet on page 143, and think through the answers to the questions that follow. Then use the information in the next section to design your own personalized weight-training plan.

Evaluating Your Muscle Strength and Endurance

1. *Modified push-ups:* Lie facedown on the floor. Place your hands next to your shoulders, knees on the floor. Push

yourself up so that you are supporting your weight on your hands and knees (see illustration below). Then, keeping your spine straight, slowly lower yourself again until your chest is only a few inches from the floor. Do as many of these as you can in one minute, and then write down the number on your worksheet. Most women will probably do between ten and twenty. If you can easily do thirty or more, try doing them from your feet (usually called a full or military-style push-up). This gives you a general idea of your *upper body strength*.

2. *Single leg squat:* Stand facing a full-length mirror. Place a chair about six inches behind the back of your legs. Lift your right knee slightly in front of you, with your foot several inches off the ground. Balance on your left leg, with your left hand *lightly* resting on a solid support, like a table or desk. (This is simply to help you maintain your balance and shouldn't be used to help support your weight!) Slowly

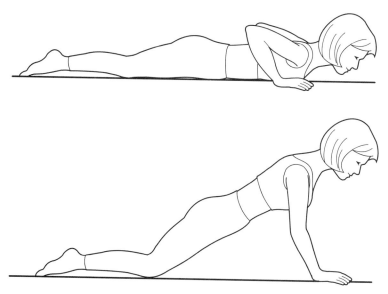

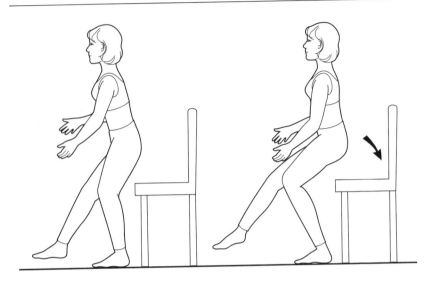

bend your knee and lower your body as if you were planning to sit down in the chair . . . but stop when you are a few inches above the chair, and slowly stand up again (see illustration above). See how many times you can complete this single leg squat. (If you're doing it correctly and have average leg strength, you will probably do less than ten.) In fact, many women can't do more than two or three of these. Now switch, and see how many you can do while balanced on the right leg. This gives you a general idea of your *lower body strength*. It may also give you an idea that you need to work on your balance!

Incidentally, don't be surprised if you find that one side is significantly stronger than the other. Right-handed women tend to have a stronger right leg; left-handed women usually have a stronger left leg. Don't forget to record your results!

3. *Crunches:* Lie down on your back. Bend your knees, plant your feet firmly on the floor, and curl up until your shoulder blades clear the floor. You can do this with your hands placed behind your head or neck, or crossed

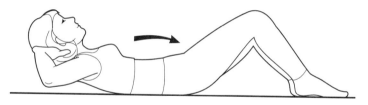

over your chest (see illustration above). Use your abdominal muscles to pull yourself up, and be sure that you aren't pulling on your neck or head with your hands. Most women using good form will be able to do at least twenty of these in one minute. Again, record your personal results on your worksheet. This gives you a good idea of your *abdominal muscle strength and endurance.*

Despite good intentions, many people unintentionally "cheat" when they do these exercises, particularly crunches. This is because they begin what I call "swinging": moving too quickly, just letting their momentum do the work. *It is better to do just a few with good form than to do many with poor form.* Remember, you cannot design an effective program for improving your health if you are not being honest with yourself about your current abilities.

DO YOU NEED MUSCLE STRENGTH OR ENDURANCE?

When we think of the work done by our muscles, many of us don't realize the difference between muscular strength and muscular endurance. *Strength* refers to the absolute force our muscle can produce upon demand, whereas *endurance* indicates the muscle's ability to perform the same motion repeatedly. Both of these are important: Imagine having the strength to hit a powerful tennis serve, but not enough muscular stamina to continue swinging the racket throughout an entire match. Or having the muscular endurance to ride a bike for 25 miles but no strength to power you up the hill to your house. Weight training does improve both strength and endurance, but subtle choices in your weight-training program will allow you to focus on one more than the other.

LET'S GET MOVING!

Patients often bring in the latest celebrity-endorsed strength-training program, asking if I think it's a good plan to follow. Some of these plans are reasonable, but many make absurd claims about their "revolutionary" fat-burning, body-sculpting secrets. Many also claim that if you follow all the exercises suggested, and do them in a particular order, you will achieve the physique of your dreams in as little as six weeks. If it were that easy, we'd be a nation of sculpted gods and goddesses! Besides just being silly, there are significant problems with this false advertising. First, the specific exercises may not be appropriate for every individual. Second, it encourages you to believe that there is some magical combination of exercises that you must follow to get good results. The truth is that essentially all strength-training exercises are effective—you just need to do them! And *you* are the single most qualified person to design a program that fits into your life.

The following guidelines can serve as the framework for your strength-training program. Think of the different exercise examples as if they were an assortment of recipe ingredients. You will have some favorite basic staples, and others that you use for variety. Mix and match them to personalize your program. There are countless different exercises and variations, so don't limit yourself to the examples included in this book. An enormous number of videos, books, and magazine articles are available to demonstrate a wide range of effective exercises. Consult the resources section at the back of this book for some suggestions. Once you become familiar with a few basic principles, it will be easy to tailor a program that will work for you.

It's Not Just *What* You Do, But *How* You Do It

When you are performing the exercises in your strength-training program, it's a great idea to do them in front of a mirror so you can check your form. You should be facing straight ahead, eyes forward and head level. Your chin should not be jutting forward, as this will strain your neck. Shoulders should be back with your posture upright. If you're standing, your knees should be ever so slightly bent (to keep you from "locking" them). Always be sure you're lifting and lowering the weight in a slow, steady motion, not swinging it up and down. Choose a weight that is heavy enough to be challenging, but light enough that you can lift it repetitively without sacrificing your good form. Women tend to be weaker in their upper bodies than in their lower bodies, so don't be surprised to find that you need a much lighter weight for your arm and shoulder exercises than for your leg exercises.

Once you put together the building blocks for your strength-training program, you can choose to do the entire set of exercises in one session, or you can break it into smaller sessions. Some options include:

- Performing the entire strength-training program two or three days a week
- Targeting the upper-body muscles in one session and the lower-body muscles in another

- Focusing on just one or two muscles in any single exercise session.

You can do your chosen exercises in any order you'd like, but if you're doing all your exercises in one session, it's a good idea to start with the largest muscles first, while you have the most energy. Warm up for at least a few minutes before you start your weight training. You can simply walk briskly for a few minutes prior to beginning your exercises, or you can weight train after your cardiovascular exercise session. Just be sure you're not too tired to maintain good form while you're lifting!

TARGETING A "PROBLEM AREA" WITH STRENGTH TRAINING

It's perfectly okay to focus on one area of your body more than others, but don't neglect any muscle group completely. For instance, if you could do only a few push-ups but had no problems with the same number of one-legged squats, you may choose to do lower extremity strengthening just once or twice a week, and focus on your arms and shoulders three times a week. However, don't make the mistake of thinking you can "spot reduce" by weight training. Focusing on one particular body part will not help you to lose fat from that spot! One of the most common myths among my patients is that doing abdominal exercises like crunches or sit-ups will result in a flat, toned stomach. Abdominal-strengthening exercises are vitally important for helping you develop core strength, but all the abdominal crunches in the world won't get rid of a potbelly! Strength training can aid in weight loss, but it needs to be combined with cardiovascular activity and a healthy diet to be most successful.

THE FITNESS FACTORS APPLIED TO STRENGTH TRAINING

Before we get started, let's define a couple of common terms. Lifting a weight once is called a *repetition* ("rep" for short). Several repetitions grouped together are called a *set*. So if you lift a weight ten times, you have just completed one set of ten repetitions. Got it? Now let's apply the five fitness factors to design your personal strength-training program.

1. Type of Activity

These days, there are a lot of options for weight-training activities. You can weight train with machines, free weights (dumbbells and barbells), or exercise bands and balls. All of these are effective ways to improve fitness and can be done at home or in a gym. If you plan to do your weight-training routine at home, invest in a guide such as *Strong Women Stay Young* or in an instructional weight-training video guide. The experts at collagevideo.com (see Resources at the end of this book) would be happy to recommend one based on your individual tastes and needs.

If you have never weight trained and you plan to join a gym, you may want to start with machines rather than free weights. This is because free weights are unsupported and generally require a bit more skill to use. It's perfectly okay, however, to begin with free weights if you prefer. If you like the social aspects of exercise, check out the strength training classes at your local fitness centers. Often termed body sculpting, these classes incorporate resistance exercises in a variety of creative ways.

Many women choose to start with a basic form of weight training called *priority training*. This means starting with one exercise and performing two or three sets of that particular exercise before moving on to the next one (with a thirty- to ninety-second rest period between sets). To design such a program for yourself, choose:

1. A minimum of eight to ten exercises for your entire program (remember, you don't have to do them all in one session).
2. At least one (and not more than two) exercise(s) for each major muscle. These are the arms (biceps in front, triceps in back), shoulders (deltoids), chest (pectoral muscles), upper and lower back (lats, rhomboids), hips and thighs (adductors in the inner thigh, abductors on the outer thigh, quadriceps in front, hamstrings in back), calves, and abdominals.
3. A minimum of six to eight and a maximum of fifteen repetitions per exercise.
4. A minimum of one and a maximum of three sets (remember, a set is one series of repetitions).

To build endurance: Choose a lighter weight and more repetitions (twelve to fifteen); begin with two days a week and work up to two to four days a week.

To build strength: Choose a heavier weight and fewer repetitions (six to eight) at least one day a week, in addition to endurance exercises two days a week.

When you are putting your individualized program together, try to incorporate some exercises such as push-ups and squats that target several muscles at once. These are some of the most effective exercises you can do because they mimic some of the demands we place on our bodies daily. Several mothers of toddlers have told me what a tremendous difference such exercises have made in helping them keep up with their active youngsters! And these busy mothers have been especially aware of another benefit of such "multi-muscle" strengthening exercises: They take very little time.

And don't exclude important *core strengthening* exercises from your plan. Targeted at the lower back muscles and abdominals, these exercises are designed to help you develop a strong, stable torso, or core. Spending just a few minutes each week training these muscles will help you avoid back pain, improve your posture, and make daily tasks a breeze.

Examples of strength-training exercises to choose from:

Arms (using free weights, bands, or machines)
biceps curl or hammer curl, cable curls
triceps kick-back or overhead extension, cable press-downs (dips will work the triceps using body weight, no other equipment necessary)

Shoulders (using free weights, bands, or machines)
side raises, overhead press, anterior (front) raises

Chest (using free weights, bands, or machines)
chest press, bench press, flies (multiple variations)

Upper back (using free weights, bands, or machines)
upright or seated row, bent row, gravitron pull-ups, lat pull-downs (do not pull down behind your head; this move also works the biceps)

Hips/Legs (using free weights, bands, or machines)
squats, leg press, lunges, hamstring curls, leg extensions, abduction (outer thighs), adduction (inner thighs), leg raises, calf raises for lower leg

Abdomen
multiple variations on crunches, back extensions

Examples of exercises that work several muscles at once
push-ups (chest, arms, shoulders)
bench press (chest, arms, shoulders)
squats (legs and buttocks)

WHEN IT COMES TO HITTING THE WEIGHTS, HEIGHT MATTERS

For the woman of average height, choosing between weight machines and free weights is purely a matter of preference. But for shorter women (5'2" or under) like me, free weights may be the wiser choice. That's because the typical weight machine at the gym is built to be used by an exerciser the height of the average man, who is three or four inches taller than the average woman. The machine's adjustments allow someone a few inches shorter than this still to be able to use the machine with good form, but beyond that, unnecessary strain can be placed on the joints. Two such examples are the leg curl machine, which can cause the shorter exerciser to place unnecessary stress on the back, and the chest press machine, whose handles can be too far apart for the more petite woman to grasp comfortably, placing more stress on the elbows and shoulders. If you want to use a particular machine but it doesn't feel comfortable, ask a fitness instructor at the gym if the machine can be modified, such as with extra pads, to improve the fit.

2. Intensity

Since intensity is basically a reflection of effort, the intensity of your weight-training program will primarily be decided by whether you focus more on exercises for muscular endurance (less intense) or those for muscular strength (more intense). To decide how intensively you plan to weight train, you need to think about your specific health goals. Most women should aim for a combination of muscle endurance and muscle-strengthening exercises. For instance, if weight training appeals to you for its metabolism-boosting weight-loss benefits, you need to be sure to include weight-training exercises that build strength, not just endurance. This means lifting heavier weights at least once a week. Lifting a more challenging weight will help you to build a bit more muscle mass, which will help incinerate calories.

3 and 4. Duration and Frequency

Muscles need a chance to recover from the challenges of strength training, so it's important to allow them enough rest time. Don't work the same muscle two days in a row, and never work any muscle more than three days in a week. If you are beginning weight training after the age of thirty-five, or are lifting heavier weights with the goal of building strength in addition to endurance, your muscles may require a slightly longer recovery period, so you may want to start with just two days a week of weight training. Be honest with yourself about how much time you are willing to spend, and how often. Can you make a commitment of twenty to thirty minutes two or three days a week? How about fifteen minutes four days a week? If you can't make that minimum time commitment, you are unlikely to see a significant response to your new weight-training program. Look back at your health goals. Aren't they worth an extra hour a week?

WEIGHT TRAINING AND HIGH BLOOD PRESSURE

The primary exception to the rule regarding strength-training intensity is the woman with heart disease or high blood pressure. Weight training in the person with cardiovascular disease is a still a subject of debate among many doctors. For years, doctors thought that patients with high blood pressure *shouldn't* lift weights at all. This was based on studies of male weight lifters, whose blood pressure went *up* to very high levels when they strained to lift a heavy weight. We learned that lifting a *very heavy* weight and holding your breath made this blood pressure elevation more likely to happen. This created concern that weight training could potentially precipitate an acute episode of dangerously high blood pressure.

Recent research, however, has shown that lifting lighter weights has a positive effect, helping to lower blood pressure. Currently, many sports medicine doctors think that lifting lighter weights for muscle endurance is a good idea for patients with *controlled* high blood pressure. The bottom line? If you have heart disease or high blood pressure, you will need to talk weight training over with your doctor. Even if your blood pressure is well controlled with medication, it's important to talk to your doctor before beginning this program, as some blood pressure medications interfere with the body's response to exercise. And *under no circumstances* should you start a weight-training program, even with light weights, if your blood pressure is not less than 160/100. If your blood pressure is this high, you will need to reduce it through other methods before you approach weight training.

Once your doctor gives you the green light to weight train, it's best to start with a weight that you're comfortable lifting, one that's no more than half of the heaviest one you can possibly lift. Pay close attention to breathing with each repetition, and avoid holding your breath. Humming, repeating a phrase (try "You can do it!"), or counting out loud while you lift weights is a good way to ensure that you keep breathing.

5. Progression

If you choose to begin weight training two days a week, a simple way to progress your program is to increase to three days each week. Alternatively, if you choose to start with lighter weights and endurance exercises, you can progress by lifting heavier weights for strength gains one day each week. And a great way to progress your program is to make a change.

Ultimately, you will get the best results by performing a variety of different weight training exercises. There are several reasons why this is the case. First, variety prevents boredom, and if strength training remains fresh and exciting, you're more likely to stick with your commitment to exercise. Second, muscles adapt quickly to new challenges. The upside of this fast response is that you'll see positive changes in your muscles soon after beginning your new program; the downside is that your progress can quickly reach a plateau. By varying your choices of exercises, you maximize the muscle's response to weight training.

And last but not least, variety can help to prevent injury. For instance, the overhead press is an exercise that effectively strengthens the *deltoid,* the large muscle in the shoulder. However, done too repetitively, this movement can injure the four small muscles in the shoulder known as the *rotator cuff.* By alternating the overhead press with a different exercise such as a front raise, this risk can be reduced. Spending time working on small muscles like those that compose the rotator cuff is also a good way to add variety while reducing risk of injury.

SAMPLE STRENGTH-TRAINING EXERCISES

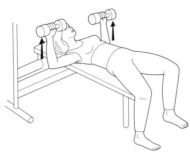

Dumbbell Chest Press

1. Hold the dumbbells shoulder-width apart above your chest. Elbows should be level with shoulders, as shown.
2. Straighten your arms, pressing the dumbbells toward the ceiling, but be sure not to lock out the elbows.
3 Slowly return to starting position.
4. Perform 2 to 3 sets, 12 to 15 reps each.

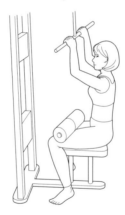

Lat Pull-Down (Upper Back)

1. Sit in front of the lat pull-down machine.
2. Hold the bar (hands shoulder-width apart) with your palms facing away, as shown.
3. Pull down until the bar almost touches your upper chest.
4. Pause, then slowly release the weight.
5. Perform 2 to 3 sets, 12 to 15 reps each.

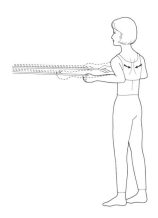

Upper Back

1. Attach some rubber tubing to a solid object.
2. Grasp the ends, keeping your arms straight ahead.
3. Squeeze your shoulder blades together and pull your arms straight back at about chest level, as shown.
4. Pause and slowly return your arms to the starting position.
5. Perform 2 to 3 sets, 12 to 15 reps each.

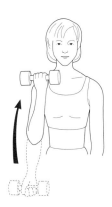

Biceps Curls

1. Hold dumbbell in one hand with your arm at your side, as shown.
2. Slowly bend your elbow, bringing the weight to your shoulder.
3. Keep your wrist straight throughout the entire movement.
4. Pause and slowly lower.
5. Perform 12 to 15 reps.
6. Switch arms.
7. Perform 2 to 3 sets on each side.

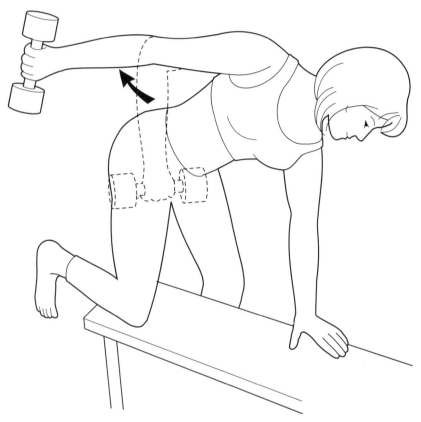

Triceps Kick-Backs

1. Place your left hand and right knee on the bench and your left foot flat on the floor, as shown.
2. Grip a dumbbell in your right hand and hold your arm at a 90-degree angle.
3. Extend your elbow straight back.
4. Pause, then slowly return the arm to the starting position.
5. Perform 12 to 15 reps.
6. Switch arms.
7. Perform 2 to 3 sets on each side.

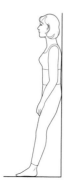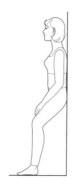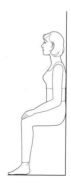

Quadriceps

1. Stand with your back against a wall. Keep your feet shoulder-width apart and about 18 inches from the wall.
2. Slowly slide down the wall until you are in a position as though you're sitting in a chair. Be sure not to let your knees go past your toes.
3. Hold 10 seconds. Repeat 10 times.
4. Try to work up to holding this position for 30 to 60 seconds.

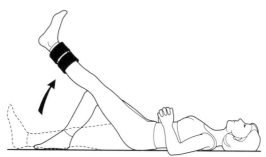

Alternate Quadriceps Exercise

1. Lie on your back with the left knee straight and the right knee bent, as shown.
2. Keeping the left leg straight, raise it so your knees are level.
3. Hold 5 seconds and slowly lower.
4. Perform 12 to 15 reps.
5. Switch legs.
6. Perform 2 to 3 sets each side.

Note: If this is too easy, add an ankle weight. Begin with 2 pounds and progress as you can.

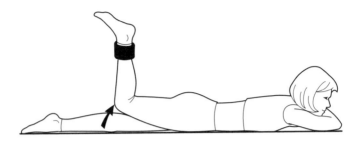

Buttocks/Hamstrings

1. Lie on your stomach with your right knee bent.
2. Raise your thigh off the floor, pressing your foot toward the ceiling.
3. Hold for 5 seconds. Slowly lower.
4. Perform 12 to 15 reps each.
5. Switch legs.
6. Perform 2 to 3 sets on each side.

Note: If this is too easy, add an ankle weight. Begin with 2 pounds and progress as you can.
(An alternate exercise for the hamstring is to keep the thigh on the floor and bend the knee, pulling the heel toward the buttock).

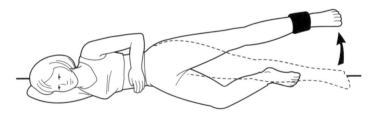

Outer Thigh

1. Lie on your right side with your right (bottom) leg slightly bent and the left (top) leg straight.
2. Raise the left leg straight up. Be sure not to let your left hip come forward.
3. Pause and slowly lower.
4. Perform 12 to 15 reps each.
5. Switch legs.
6. Perform 2 to 3 sets on each side.

Note: If this is too easy, add an ankle weight. Begin with 2 pounds and progress as you can.

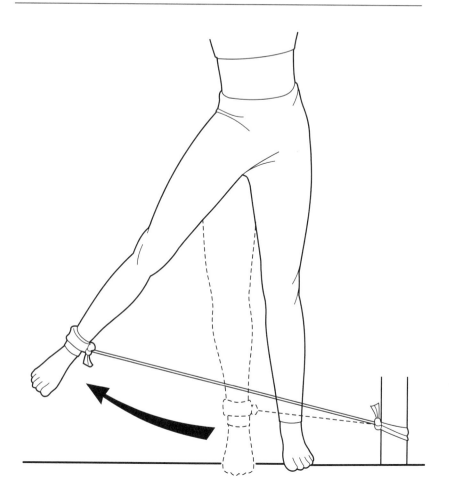

Alternate Outer Thigh Exercise

1. Attach one end of some rubber tubing to a solid object and the other end to the right ankle, as shown.
2. Stand straight with your hand resting against a table or wall for support.
3. Keeping the right leg straight, raise it out to the side from the hip.
4. Hold 3 to 5 seconds, slowly release.
5. Do 12 to 15 reps.
6. Switch legs.
7. Perform 2 to 3 sets each side.

Note: You can also perform this exercise with a weight instead of tubing.

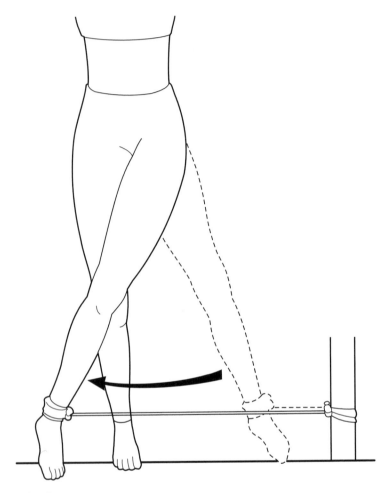

Inner Thigh

1. Attach one end of some rubber tubing to a solid object and the other end to the left ankle, as shown.
2. Stand straight with your hand resting against a table or wall for support.
3. Keeping your left leg straight, toe pointed, pull it in front of your right leg.
4. Hold 3 to 5 seconds, slowly release.
5. Do 12 to 15 reps.
6. Switch legs.
7. Perform 2 to 3 sets each side.

Note: You can also perform this exercise with a weight instead of tubing.

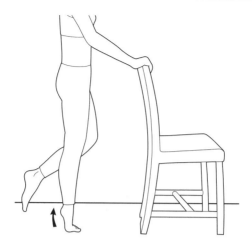

Calves

1. Stand on your right leg holding on to a chair as shown. Left foot should be off the floor.
2. Slowly rise up onto the ball of your right foot, feeling the right calf muscle contract.
3. Pause, then slowly lower to the floor.
4. Perform 12 to 15 reps.
5. Switch legs.
6. Perform 2 to 3 sets each side.

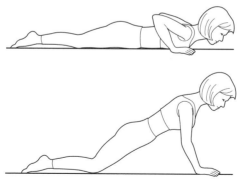

Modified Push-ups

1. Lie on your stomach, hands flat and arms bent at your side as shown.
2. Straightening your arms while keeping your knees on the floor, push your torso off the floor.
3. Hold 2 to 3 seconds, then slowly lower.
4. Repeat 10 to 20 times.

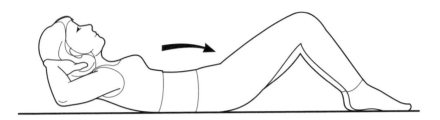

Crunches/Abdominals

1. Lie on your back with your knees bent.
2. Place your hands behind your head to support the neck.
3. Tighten your stomach and slowly raise your head and shoulders off the floor. Be sure not to pull or strain your neck. Keep your eyes focused on the ceiling.
4. Pause and slowly lower.
5. Perform 20 to 30 repetitions slowly.

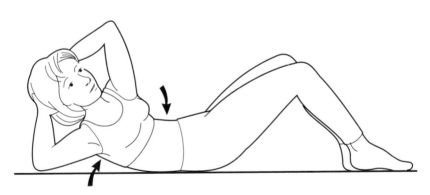

Alternative Crunches (Obliques—Sides of Abdominals)

1. Lie on your back with your knees bent.
2. Place your hands behind your head to support the neck.
3. Raise your head and shoulders off the floor and curl your left elbow toward your right knee as shown.
4. Pause and slowly lower.
5. Repeat in the opposite direction.
6. Perform 10 to 20 repetitions on each side.

OTHER CONSIDERATIONS WHEN DESIGNING YOUR STRENGTH-TRAINING PLAN

Consideration	Possible Choice
Your goal is weight loss.	Weight-training program for both the upper and lower body three days a week.
Osteoporosis prevention is a concern.	Add balance training exercises like tai chi.
You have high blood pressure.	If your blood pressure is controlled (140/90 or less), and your doctor has given you the green light, begin with lower weights (40 to 50 percent of the heaviest you can lift).
	If your blood pressure is between 140/90 and 160/100, check with your doctor before beginning weight training.
	If your blood pressure is 160/100 or more, do not begin weight training—work with your doctor on getting it lower through other means.
You want to exercise at home.	Strength-training videotapes; bands or free weights; exercises like push-ups, squats, and dips that require little or no equipment.
You want to exercise with a partner.	Taking classes at a gym; finding an exercise buddy to weight train with; hiring a personal trainer.
You have an injury or joint pain.	See a doctor for diagnosis and treatment before beginning weight training.
You are "pear-shaped" (thighs wider than hips).	Focusing on strength-training exercises for the chest, back, and shoulders can help your body appear more balanced.

YOUR WEIGHT-TRAINING CHECKLIST

1. Be sure to go through a full range of motion as you perform each exercise.

2. Pay attention to your posture and form. Lift and lower the weight during each repetition, don't swing it! Using good form, you should need about two to four seconds to lift the weight, and another two to four seconds to lower it.

3. Don't forget to breathe! Many weight lifting experts say that the most natural way to breathe is to inhale as you lower the weight and exhale as you lift it. The "right" way is whatever works for you, as long as you aren't holding your breath. Holding your breath increases your blood pressure and can make you feel light-headed, or can even cause you to faint.

4. Keep your abdominal muscles contracted during each lift.

5. If you're a beginner, start with one set, then work up to three. While you are learning technique, it is makes sense to choose a lighter weight and a higher number of repetitions. So you might start an exercise using five pounds and performing one set of fifteen repetitions, and work your way up to three sets of eight to ten repetitions using a ten-pound weight.

6. Rest for thirty to sixty seconds between sets; rest for a minute or two between different exercises. If you rest longer than that, you will lose some of the cardiovascular benefit of weight training.

7. When you can complete all the sets of one exercise with good form, and your muscles are not fatigued, increase the amount of weight for that exercise. If you can't do the same number of sets with the heavier weight, try doing two sets with the lighter weight and one with the heavier; increase slowly as you get stronger.

8. After your workout, make a note of how much weight you used for each exercise. Over time, this is something you probably won't have to do, but when you're a beginner, it's often helpful to have a reference for your next session.

WRITE IT DOWN

Keeping the five fitness factors in mind, complete the worksheet below. This will be Part Three of your personal exercise program. Plan to follow it for the first four weeks, although remember, it is *your* exercise program: you can change any of the fitness factors at any time. Use the samples in the next few pages for suggestions, but use your knowledge of yourself to design a program that will work for you.

Part Three of My Personal Exercise Program

Muscular Strength and Endurance

Results of my first assessment:
modified push-ups
crunches
single leg squats

Weight training exercises I plan to start with, and where:

Time I plan to spend at each weight-training session:

Frequency I plan to weight train (mark these days on your calendar!):

My strength and muscular endurance goals include:

My health goals include:

To help stay motivated, I will:

SAMPLE STRENGTH-TRAINING PROGRAMS

#1: Louise

> Louise, a forty-two-year-old nurse, wanted to lower her high blood pressure.

Louise's Personal Strength-Training Program

Results of first fitness assessment: Louise could do very few single leg squats, fifteen crunches, and eleven modified push-ups.

Activity: Louise felt that she would enjoy the camaraderie of a body-sculpting class, but she didn't want to pay the cost of a gym membership just for a couple of classes a week. She circulated a proposal at work and found several other nurses and hospital employees who were also interested in such a class. She recruited the exercise physiologist from the hospital's cardiac rehabilitation program to lead the class.

Intensity level: Because of her high blood pressure, Louise chose endurance exercises with light weights.

Duration: Forty-five-minute body-sculpting classes.

Frequency: Twice a week.

To progress: After eight weeks, she began to alternate resistance bands with light weights, and added push-ups and sit-ups at home twice a week.

Her first fitness goals: To complete an entire forty-five-minute class.

Her health goal: To lower her blood pressure.

To help stay motivated: Louise left fitness clothes and shoes in her locker at work so she could just switch from her uniform to exercise gear. Exercising with her colleagues gave her a real motivational boost.

#2: Karen

Karen, a thirty-five-year-old attorney, took aerobic dance classes but was frustrated by her inability to lose weight.

Karen's Strength-Training Program

Results of first fitness assessment: Karen was amazed to find that although she could do quite a few single leg squats, she could do very few crunches without cheating, and only six modified push-ups.

Activity: Karen chose to combine weight training with free weights and machines. Her chosen exercises were biceps curl machine, triceps cable press-downs, lat pull-downs, anterior deltoid raises, dumbbell flies, leg press machine, hamstring curl machine, and abdominal crunches.

Intensity level: Karen chose a combination of endurance and strengthening exercises.

Duration: Twenty-minute weight training sessions.

Frequency: Endurance exercises twice a week (three sets of ten repetitions), strength training with heavier weights once a week (two sets of eight repetitions).

To progress: After six weeks, she began to modify her new routine, adding new exercises such as push-ups and squats.

Her first fitness goals: To complete two sets of ten modified push-ups.

Her health goal: Weight loss.

To help stay motivated: Karen hired a personal trainer once a month to help her plan new exercises so she wouldn't get bored.

#3: Margaret

Sixty-four-year-old Margaret wanted to reduce her risk of osteoporosis.

Margaret's Personal Strength-Training Program

Results of first fitness assessment: Margaret could do seven single leg squats on the right, but only three on the left, and she had trouble keeping her balance while doing them. She could do twelve crunches and three modified push-ups.

Activity: Margaret chose to weight train at home with a combination of free weights and resistance bands. Her chosen exercises were standing leg lifts for both inner and outer thighs, standing hamstring curls, biceps curl, triceps kickbacks, upright row, and dumbbell flies. She also joined a Saturday-morning tai chi class at a local community center to work on her balance. She chose to stand rather than sit for as many exercises as possible in order to maximize the weight-bearing benefit of each exercise.

Intensity level: A combination of endurance, strengthening, and balance exercises.

Duration: Twenty-minute weight training sessions (two sets, ten repetitions), forty-five-minute tai chi class.

Frequency: Weight-training exercises at home two days weekly, and a tai chi class once a week.

To progress: Margaret added modified wall squats and push-ups to her routine. She began subscribing to a couple of women's health and fitness magazines, which gave her new ideas for varying her exercise program.

Her first fitness goal: To complete ten single leg squats on each side without losing her balance.

Her health goal: Reduce her risk of osteoporosis.

To help stay motivated: Margaret found that she had more energy and was able to keep up with her husband on weekend hikes, which kept her motivated to continue.

WHAT CAN *YOU* EXPECT FROM A STRENGTH-TRAINING PROGRAM?

If you consistently follow the program you've created for yourself, you will begin to see results in as little as four weeks. You can expect the following:

What you should see: Developing muscles in four to eight weeks; improved posture.

What you should feel: Post-exercise soreness decreases after the first two weeks; arms and legs feel firmer; clothing feels looser; energy and stamina increase.

What you should expect: Loss of one to two pounds of fat in four to six weeks and a corresponding gain of one pound of muscle (so the scale may not change!). After three months, on average, you will have lost four to five pounds of fat and gained three pounds of muscle, for a net weight loss of one to two pounds. Your daily calorie use will be increased by 10 to 15 percent.

What you can expect if you do this for one year: A gain of five or more pounds of muscle and a loss of ten or more pounds of fat; firmer arms and legs; a smaller dress size; an increase of at least 50 percent in strength; stronger muscles and bones; improved exercise and sports performance; ease with everyday tasks such as carrying bags and opening jars or heavy doors. Your cholesterol level and blood pressure should drop by several points. If you stick with this program, you will decrease your risk of osteoporosis, heart disease, diabetes, high blood pressure, and obesity.

What you should watch out for: Don't forget to make periodic adjustments in your routine to prevent boredom and limitation of muscle adaptation. Be aware that lifting too little weight will limit your potential gains, and the lack of results will ruin your motivation. However, trying to lift too much weight will also ruin your motivation, because it will be too uncomfortable and discouraging. And it will increase your risk of injury. Fight the temptation to do only the exercises you like or find easy. We all have a tendency to emphasize our strengths and ignore our weaknesses, but giving in to this will prevent you from making maximal gains.

NO PAIN, NO GAIN?

Many women will complete their first weight-training session filled with energy and pride—only to wake up the next morning so stiff and sore they don't want to get out of bed. Such soreness is called *delayed onset muscle soreness,* or DOMS, because it occurs at least six hours after the exercise session. Don't panic: To some degree, it's to be expected, and it will get less frequent as you and your exercise routine get better acquainted.

What Is DOMS?

Many people, including athletes and fitness trainers, will tell you this is lactic acid buildup in the muscles you've been using—but they're wrong! Lactic acid does develop when we exercise, but it's gone from the muscle within a couple of hours of stopping activity, long before DOMS sets in. So what really happens to cause the soreness known as DOMS? As you lift and lower a weight, tiny tears known as *microtears* occur in the muscle fibers. These affect just a few of the muscle fibers in any specific muscle. The body's response to these "injuries" of the muscle fibers is to send in a cleanup crew of white blood cells to repair the microtears in the muscles. While they're working, the white blood cells release various chemicals that cause inflammation and swelling in the muscle tissue. This, then, is what you feel the next morning when you crawl out of bed.

How Can You Minimize DOMS?

First, start your weight-training program slowly. Beginning gradually will give your muscles time to adapt to new demands. And be encouraged by the fact that muscles have an amazing memory: they adapt to these microtears through a variety of ways that leave them less sore after each workout.

What Can You Do If You Have DOMS?

The truth is that although many remedies will be suggested, nothing works like a tincture of time. Topical medications, non-steroidal anti-inflammatory drugs (NSAIDs) like ibuprofen, aspirin, massage, heat, and ice are all popular forms of treatments against DOMS. Try one of them if you like, but remember, the best treatment is prevention: Start exercising gradually. Your muscles will thank you for it!

And remember, as your muscles adapt to exercise over a couple of weeks, the soreness will gradually decrease and then stop occurring. Some women think this means they are no longer making fitness gains (the "no pain, no gain" concept). But don't worry: no pain just means that your muscles have adapted to the demands of your training program, and that you are more fit than you were when you began.

DO I NEED A PERSONAL TRAINER?

This is probably the most common question I'm asked by women beginning a weight-training program. To decide if you need a personal trainer, ask yourself the following three questions:

- Am I feeling intimidated by the thought of starting a weight-training program?
- Am I feeling unsure of how to do the exercises correctly?
- Am I more likely to stay committed to weight training if I work with a personal trainer?

If you answered yes to two or more of these questions, hiring a personal trainer to help you get going may be a good idea.

How to Find a Good Personal Trainer

If you've decided that you would benefit from one-on-one instruction, the next step is to find the right personal trainer for you. But beware: Although the number of personal trainers in the United States has skyrocketed in the past decade, many of them have no respectable credentials and no experience training women who are novice exercisers. As personal training has become big business, there has been no corresponding standard national credentialing process. There are some very impressive-sounding "fitness associations" that, upon closer inspection, turn out to be all glitz with no substance. For instance, one such association offers "certification" to anyone who pays a fee to take its online true-false exam. Compare that to the American College of Sports Medicine's rigorous process, in which prospective trainers are required to take a six-hour written and practical exam.

Many of the patients I see work with personal trainers, and when I ask about certification the answers I often hear are:

"The trainer was recommended by my friend."
"The trainer works at my gym."
"S/he is really nice."
"S/he seems really good."

The irony is that those women with the least weight training experience stand to gain the most from a personal trainer, but have the least knowledge in determining a potential trainer's qualifications.

If *you* want to hire a personal trainer, do some sleuthing to find one:

- with respectable credentials, such as certification by the American College of Sports Medicine (ACSM), American Council on Exercise (ACE), or the National Strength and Conditioning Association
- with experience working with other women like you (with your medical concerns, past experience, goals, etc.)
- who encourages and answers your questions
- who makes you feel comfortable
- who sticks to training and doesn't push you to buy or use supplements

STRENGTH TRAINING AND A HIGH PROTEIN DIET

A common myth in strength-training circles is that in order to achieve results, you must switch to a diet that's high in protein. This is simply not true. Your muscles need all three of the basic components of food: protein, carbohydrates, and fat. Protein forms the building blocks of muscle tissue and is the raw material used for muscles' repair process, which requires only a few ounces of dietary protein each day. For energy, the muscles' fuel of choice is carbohydrate, and fat is the runner-up! So it takes all three to keep your muscles healthy and active. If you're still concerned, it's perfectly okay to add a bit more protein to your daily intake, but most women's diets already have all the protein their muscles need.

MAKING YOUR HEALTH AND FITNESS DREAMS COME TRUE

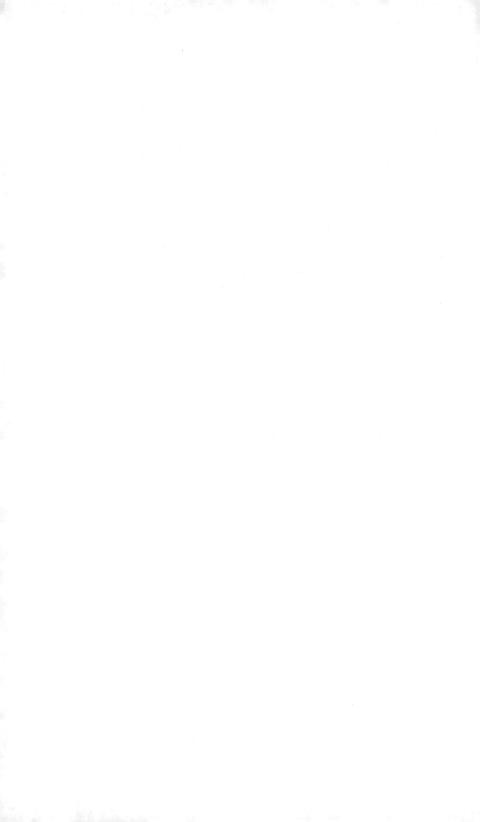

CHAPTER 6

DOES YOUR FITNESS PLAN HAVE STAYING POWER?

FOR MANY WOMEN, *beginning* an exercise program is the hardest part. But for others, sticking with exercise is the real challenge. Research shows that most people who are going to drop an exercise program do so within four weeks, whereas women who stay committed to an exercise program for one hundred days are much more likely to continue exercise long-term. This is one of the reasons it is crucial that you develop a plan you can stick with. Creating a permanent place in your week for exercise means making it a habit, like brushing your teeth or washing your hair. But it also means periodically reassessing your exercise routine to be sure it's not *too much* of a habit: making occasional changes in your fitness plan is imperative to maximize your results and attain your goals. And that's where the fifth fitness factor, *progression*, really comes into play.

One of the most common mistakes I see among women who exercise is performing the same routine over and over again. While repetition is a great way to master a new skill, constantly performing the same exercises prevents you from reaping all the rewards of fitness. Worse, it contributes to boredom, loss of motivation, and injury. But periodically altering your fitness plan minimizes these risks.

TAKING YOUR FITNESS TO THE NEXT LEVEL

If you've been exercising for at least four to six weeks, it's time to evaluate the progress you've made so far. Look back at pages 65, 93, 143 and the results of your first fitness assessments, then try taking the self-evaluations for cardiovascular health, flexibility, and muscular fitness again. This gives you a chance to see, in concrete measures, how exercise has positively impacted your life. How much farther can you walk or run in ten minutes? Are your hamstrings more flexible? Can you do more push-ups? Do you feel more alert? Do you have more energy, better posture, lower blood pressure? Congratulate yourself on each gain, no matter how modest: each represents an improvement in at least one aspect of your health!

Now that you have mastered the basics of cardiovascular exercise, flexibility, and weight training, you're ready to learn how to continue individualizing and progressing your fitness plan for life. We'll do this through a series of techniques designed to help you:

- fight boredom
- remain committed
- troubleshoot, if you're not getting the results you anticipated
- reassess, to make sure you're meeting your goals
- conquer new challenges
- stay healthy

STEPPING UP YOUR CARDIOVASCULAR FITNESS

Ellen was enjoying walking with a neighbor several mornings a week, and she reported that she was sleeping better and feeling less stressed. After eight weeks, though, she was frustrated that she had been unable to lose more than a couple of pounds.

Why wasn't Ellen seeing the weight-loss results she wanted? When we sat down to troubleshoot her lack of progress, Ellen was able to pinpoint her main obstacle quickly. Although she enjoyed the companionship of walking with her neighbor, Betty, she realized that Betty walked much more slowly than she did. In addition, Betty liked to stop and chat with other neighbors who were out gardening or sitting on their porches. Ellen was frustrated because her exercise sessions had become more about being social than getting fit, but she didn't know how to change that.

I reassured Ellen that although she wasn't losing weight, she was still getting a significant health benefit from her current level of exercise. Even her low-intensity exercise was helping to reduce the risk of many diseases, including heart disease, diabetes, and some cancers. And the weight-bearing nature of walking was a bonus for her bone health. Simply realizing that she was getting all those health benefits made Ellen feel much less discouraged and much happier about her exercise commitment. To lose weight, however, she would need to burn more calories. Ellen needed to alter one of the fitness factors. Since she wanted to keep walking as her primary activity, she needed to increase the *intensity, frequency,* or *duration* of her exercise sessions.

Ellen had several options. She could walk alone on some mornings, making those sessions more challenging, and walk with Betty on easy days, when she didn't mind the slower pace. Another alternative was to let Betty start out a few minutes ahead, so that Ellen would have to walk quickly to catch up, or to add a few extra blocks on at the end, after she'd dropped Betty off at home. Or she could begin incorporating *intervals* into her exercise session.

Interval Training

Interval training, often referred to simply as intervals, is a technique many successful athletes have used for years. But you don't have to be an elite athlete to get the metabolism-boosting benefits of this type of training. Interval training refers to the practice of alternating fast and slow periods of exercise. (The term *interval* actually refers to the slow period of exercise between the faster spurts.) Again, it's not the terminology that's important for the average exerciser to remember, it's just the concept that's important to grasp. By alternating bursts of speed with pauses, or slow activity, you can improve your cardiovascular fitness, incinerate calories, and avoid the higher risk of injury that results from a sustained, intense exercise session. Virtually *anyone* at any level of fitness can incorporate interval training into her routine.

Let's use Ellen as an example. She decided that she would start out with Betty and use the first ten minutes of their walking as a warm-up period. Then, when they reached an agreed-upon corner, Ellen would stride quickly away from Betty, increasing her heart rate until her perceived rate of exertion was about 8 on her RPE scale. She would try to continue walking at that pace for thirty seconds, then turn and walk back toward Betty at that same pace. When she reached Betty, she would slow down and resume walking with her at the slower pace, until she was ready to repeat the process. Ellen found that by adding a few of these intervals to her walking program three days each week, she began to burn more calories and achieve the weight loss she wanted.

While interval training is an excellent way to both burn calories and improve speed, it is a technique that shouldn't be used for daily workouts. The more highly trained you become, and the more intense your workout, the less frequently you should do interval training. I recommend most women stick with once a week for intervals, although if you're generally exercising at a lower intensity, like Ellen, two or three times a week is fine.

How to Incorporate Interval Training into Your Fitness Plan

No matter what your choice of activity, you can introduce the concept of interval training. You should always start with at least a five- to ten-minute warm-up period. When you're ready, increase your exercise intensity for thirty to sixty seconds of high-level activity. Then slow down to an easy speed and let your heart rate come back down until you're breathing easily again. The better shape you're in, the less time it will take for your heart rate to come down (therefore, the shorter your rest interval will need to be). When you're ready, repeat this sequence. Experiment and see what feels challenging to you. You may find that you can increase your speed for only ten or fifteen seconds, and that it takes you several minutes to be ready for the next increase in intensity. Over time, you will find that you can go faster for longer, and the time you need for recovery will decrease. Initially, aim for three or four intervals in your first few tries at this new technique, and gradually increase the number you do. Five is a good number to shoot for; don't exceed ten intervals in one training session.

Is it safe to use ankle weights while walking to burn extra calories?

No! The theory behind carrying extra weight while exercising is a simple one: The more weight you carry, the harder you have to work, so the more calories you'll burn. But carrying this extra weight by wearing ankle weights while walking or jogging can increase your risk of injury. A better idea: A weighted vest, which distributes weight more evenly and doesn't add extra strain to the ligaments, muscles, and tendons in the ankle. But remember, there's nothing magic about wearing a vest: carrying an extra ten or fifteen pounds on your torso increases the number of calories you burn by roughly 10 to 20 percent. You can achieve the same result by simply adding a few minutes to your daily walks.

BATTLE EXERCISE BOREDOM

Loren began an exercise program after her sister had a heart attack at the age of fifty-one. She joined a nearby gym, where she began riding a stationary bicycle three days each week and taking a body-sculpting class on Saturday mornings. After a couple of months, she was bored with her routine and started skipping workouts.

While the simplest solution for Loren was to stop bicycling and try a new activity, the smartest move was to evaluate why bicycling wasn't holding her interest. That would allow her to identify any mistakes that she might accidentally transfer to another activity. In fact, when Loren and I talked about her stationary cycling at the gym, several issues became apparent. She had begun riding the bike on a manual setting, using a low level of intensity. At first, that had been challenging enough, but as time passed and her level of fitness improved, it became much easier. She had begun reading while on the bike and as a result stopped following her heart rate. She wasn't aware of how much, or how little, effort she was expending. And although she liked bicycling outdoors, she was disappointed that she found the stationary bike so uninteresting.

Loren had encountered several problems common to new exercisers. Without being aware of it, she had quickly reached a *results plateau*. Instead of changing one of the fitness factors, like altering the intensity or duration of exercise, she kept following the same routine. Her muscles had gotten used to the demands of her unchanging patterns of exercise and were no longer being stimulated to improve. Reading while on the bike had been distracting her from riding vigorously, and therefore threatened the quality and results of her exercise sessions.

Loren needed to focus on getting the most out of her workouts. There were several ways she could do this, including trying a setting on the bike other than the manual one, such as the hill program or cross-country race, to engage her mind while exercising. One of the reasons she enjoyed bicycling outside was that she frequently found someone to ride with, so I suggested she try a cycling class (usually known as spinning) at her gym, which would challenge her on the bike while providing social stimulation. And to keep boredom at bay, it was a good time to spice Loren's exercise program with an introduction to *variety-training*.

Is a recumbent bike better than an old-fashioned one?
There are advantages to both designs. The recumbent bike allows you to sit upright, with your legs in front, rather than underneath, your torso. Some women simply find this position to be more comfortable than leaning forward toward the handlebars of a standard bike. One of the main differences between the two styles of bike is that the recumbent bike's seat is styled with a back. This design provides extra back support, which is popular with exercisers with chronic back pain, and has been particularly welcomed by pregnant women. However, women who have tight hamstrings may find the position of the recumbent bike actually to increase discomfort in their lower backs.

An advantage of the standard bike is that the core muscles in your abdomen and back work to support you in this position, which helps you to develop endurance in these important torso-stabilizing muscles. The standard bike also seems to be more comfortable for many women who suffer from a common knee ailment called *anterior knee pain syndrome* (see page 265).

You've Heard of Cross-Training, But What's Variety-Training?

Traditionally, cross-training is a term used in athletics to refer to a *method of training for a specific sport*. For instance, running has been used as a cross-training technique by athletes in many sports, including swimming and softball. The idea of cross-training as it applies to these athletes is that the *secondary* activity (running) will make them better at their *primary* sport (swimming or softball). Although it has never actually been proven, some also believe that cross-training in this sense will help reduce injuries.

To the general population, cross-training means something very different. It has become a term popularly used to describe an exercise program with a variety of components. For instance, a woman who swims or uses the rowing machine at the gym, hikes on weekends, and weight trains might refer to these activities as cross-training. A more accurate term is probably *variety-training*. Regardless of the terminology, variety in an exercise program has many benefits. By alternating activities, muscles are challenged in different ways. This limits the risk of injuries from repetitive use and maximizes the muscle response to training. It can also be one of the most effective ways to prevent exercise from becoming boring.

You can design your own *variety-training* program based on your personal interests and goals. Remember, though, no matter how well you've mastered one type of activity, when you start a new one, start at the beginning. Begin with twenty minutes of the new activity and gradually increase. Reapply the fitness factors, and you won't go wrong! Even if you're perfectly happy with your exercise routine, try to make some small change every few weeks. Some examples:

- If you use fitness videos, try a *different type* of video. For instance, if you've been using a step routine, consider trying a yoga, boxing, or weight training tape.
- If you exercise at a gym, try a *new machine* or a new combination of machines. For instance, if you usually walk on the treadmill, try the elliptical trainer, stair stepper, or rowing machine. Or break a thirty-minute exercise session into three ten-minute mini-workouts. For instance, follow ten minutes of

What burns more calories: the stair stepper or the treadmill?
Calories aren't burned by either of those machines—they're burned by your "human machine"! The number of calories you burn while doing any particular activity is a function of how much you weigh (the bigger you are, the more calories you use); how intensely you exercise; and how long you exercise. And whether or not you cheat. Cheating at exercise can be done through a variety of methods, with or without intent. For instance, holding on to the rails of either the treadmill or the stair stepper will decrease the number of calories you burn. Some experts believe people tend to push themselves harder on the treadmill and are more likely to cheat with other equipment, accounting for the findings of some researchers that exercisers burn more calories on the treadmill. I frequently see a woman increase the level of difficulty on a piece of equipment, then step on and use it incorrectly, unknowingly sabotaging her workout.

Always follow the rule of good form. If you aren't sure whether you're using a piece of equipment with good form, ask a trainer or your gym's fitness staff for guidance. If you can't exercise at the level you've selected without sacrificing form, lower the level of difficulty. Using proper form is critical to getting optimal results without injury.

your usual activity like treadmill walking with ten minutes on the bike, then ten minutes on the cross-country ski machine. The possibilities are endless.

- If you walk outside, *change your route* to include a hill; try adding a couple of minutes of jogging to the middle of your walk; go hiking or in-line skating.

Use the chart opposite as a guideline to start thinking about your alternate activities. What would *you* enjoy?

If you started your exercise program with:	Consider adding for variety:	Why:
Walking or jogging	Swimming	For its upper body and joint-friendly non-impact benefits
Running	Bicycling	For its non-impact benefits; and because running emphasizes the hamstring (back of the thigh), whereas bicycling emphasizes the quadriceps (front of the thigh)
Swimming	Walking, aerobic dance, kickboxing, or jogging	These weight-bearing activities will boost your bone mass
Fitness videotapes	In-line skating, walking	Both can be done without a gym and will get you outside; both are weight-bearing and therefore good for your bones; skating is non-impact

I read a magazine article that said you should choose exercises based on your body shape. I'm bottom-heavy and love the stair stepper, but the article said I should stay away from it and ride a stationary bike instead. Is that true?

No. You will not develop a heavier bottom by using any particular piece of equipment! Most women who are "bottom-heavy" just have extra fat stored in their thighs, hips, and buttocks. Any activity that you enjoy will help you burn some of those stored calories and will ultimately make you leaner. Recognize that your muscles will get a bit bigger as they become stronger and more toned, so don't be alarmed if there is a slight increase in your lower body size as you begin to get fit. As your muscles develop, they will boost your fat-burning potential; the stored fat will begin to melt away, uncovering your newly toned muscles!

Part Four of My Personal Exercise Program

Progressing Cardiovascular Fitness

Results of my first cardiovascular fitness assessment:

Results of my second cardiovascular fitness assessment:

Health goals I feel I'm meeting, or continuing to work toward:

To progress from this point, I'm going to try:

To help stay motivated, I will:

SAMPLE PROGRAM FOR PROGRESSION OF CARDIOVASCULAR EXERCISE

Melody has been exercising at the gym for three months. For cardiovascular exercise, she gradually progressed from brisk walking to jogging on the treadmill, which she does for twenty to thirty minutes three days a week. She's happy with her current exercise program, but would like to lose a few pounds before her high school reunion.

Results of first cardiovascular fitness assessment: Melody walked about half a mile in ten minutes.

Results of second cardiovascular fitness assessment: Two months after she began exercising, Melody jogged more than three-quarters of a mile in ten minutes.

The *health benefits* Melody was happy about getting from exercise were more energy, stress reduction, better sleep, enhanced bone and heart health. The additional goal she wanted to work toward was weight loss.

To progress and try to achieve her weight-loss goal, Melody decided to make two changes. First, she added interval training two days a week by building in short bursts of sprinting while jogging. Second, she added two extra days of cardiovascular exercise by joining a dance class.

To help her stay motivated, Melody stuck her high school yearbook picture on the bathroom mirror. She also picked out a dress to wear to the reunion, and hung it in the front of her closet as a daily reminder.

The stationary bike I ride at the gym gives me a report of total calories burned. Is it accurate?

Don't put too much faith in the number you see displayed on any piece of equipment! The "calories burned" feature frequently overestimates the truth by as much as 15 to 20 percent. This number is calculated by computer from a formula using the information it has: the speed, distance, and duration of your session. If it factors in your weight, you'll get a closer estimate than if it doesn't take that variable into account. But it doesn't know whether you leaned on the handlebars, chatted with a neighbor, or whether you were working as hard as you could, using terrific form. So remember that the number you see is simply an estimate. Only *you* know how hard you really worked!

A Final Note

Some fitness experts frown on reading, watching television, or even listening to music while exercising. In my opinion, this is simply one more issue that needs to be individualized. Some people don't enjoy exercise enough to do it regularly without the distraction of a good book or favorite television program. Others simply juggle so many time demands that they will skip exercise altogether if they can't do more than one thing at once. For instance, one of my friends is a busy physician with three young children. An avid exerciser, she has found that the only way she is able to fit both regular exercise and the latest medical journals into her week is to combine the two by reading while she exercises. Similarly, one of my patients is a busy politician who reads the morning paper while doing a stretching routine.

And researchers in several countries, including the United States, Great Britain, and Japan, have found that exercisers who listen to music not only enjoy exercise more, they exercise *better.* Music provides motivation and diverts attention from muscle fatigue. And studies show that music improves how quickly you master new patterns of movement. Although any music that you enjoy will help to motivate your exercise sessions, the best music is rhythmic, with a tempo that matches your target heart rate range or pace. There are walking tapes in existence that were designed specifically for this purpose, letting you choose a tempo corresponding to walking 2.5 to 3, 3 to 3.5, or 4 miles per hour. You can also make your own exercise tape or CD. If you choose to make your own, start with slower songs for your warm-up, then pick up the tempo when you're ready to pick up your pace. Add another slower set at the end for your cool-down and after-exercise stretching.

Just remember, if you combine another activity with your exercise program, don't let it monopolize your attention. This isn't hard to do, it just takes a little practice. If you read while exercising, pause at the bottom of every few pages and check your heart rate or intensity level. While watching television, consider using commercial breaks for interval training. And don't let your movement slow down if the tempo of the music you're listening to does!

MEASURING FITNESS THROUGH VO$_2$ MAX

While estimating target heart rate based on the formulas in the earlier chapters is generally adequate, you may want to take a more scientific approach, which can be done by measuring VO$_2$ max. VO$_2$ max is the maximal (max) volume (V) of oxygen (O$_2$) that can be delivered to your muscles. The higher your VO$_2$ max, the higher your level of cardiovascular fitness (also called *cardiopulmonary fitness* or *aerobic capacity*). Measuring VO$_2$ max requires exercising on a treadmill, bike, or other piece of equipment while hooked up to a sophisticated device that records the amount of oxygen and carbon dioxide you exhale. In the past, VO$_2$ max measurements were mainly limited to elite athletes or research, but today it's available in many other settings—including some health clubs. For reliability and safety reasons, this test should be administered by an exercise physiologist or similarly qualified health care professional.

BOOSTING YOUR STRENGTH-TRAINING PROGRAM

Cece had three sessions with a personal trainer to help her get started on a weight-training program. She was pleased with the muscle development she noticed after six weeks, and she felt her clothing getting looser. But as time passed, she felt the exercises were becoming less challenging. Although she gradually increased the weights the way the trainer had suggested, she didn't feel she was continuing to get results.

When Cece first came to see me, it wasn't clear why she wasn't seeing results. She showed me a list of basic weight-training exercises that the trainer had given her, and they all seemed appropriate. When we went over Cece's list of exercises one by one, however, a spotlight shown on her error: she had gradually eliminated some of the exercises she found difficult, whittling her actual strength-training program down to five exercises. She hadn't even realized this until we sat down and went over her weight-training program. As soon as Cece began incorporating the exercises she had dropped, she once again began to see results.

Cece's mistake is actually quite common. Many women tell me they don't do a particular exercise because they don't like it. What they really mean (and often, they don't even realize it) is that the exercise is difficult. All the more reason to tackle it! An exercise you find difficult is, in all likelihood, one that challenges a muscle that is particularly weak. It's human nature to ignore your weakest points and to play to your strengths. While doing so is probably an advantage in many areas of life, it's particularly detrimental when it comes to strength training. The most fit women are the ones who are willing to work on strengthening their weaknesses. *You will not maximize the results of weight training if you ignore your weaknesses.*

Once you have developed a strength-training program, remember that it's important to make periodic adjustments, just like you did with cardiovascular exercise. There is an endless variety of options for modifying your strength-training program a little, or a lot. Or you can change it entirely! It's very important that, every few weeks, you reassess your current program and goals. If you want to make a change, be specific about your reasons. Is it just to keep your muscles challenged in new ways? To combat boredom? To cut down the time your current program takes?

Once you decide what parts you'd like to change, consider the following techniques.

1. *Try circuit training.* For a beginner planning to progress her program, circuit training is a great place to start. In circuit training, you begin with one set of an exercise for a particular body part, then move quickly to complete one set of another exercise for a different body part. You use this technique to complete a full circuit of several different exercises. How many exercises you choose to do is up to you; most women choose eight to twelve different exercises. You then rest for no more than three minutes, and then repeat the circuit one or two more times. When you finish, you will have completed two or three sets of each exercise.

For instance, your circuit-training program might look like this:

One set of eight repetitions of exercise #1: bench press
One set of eight repetitions of exercise #2: quadriceps extension
One set of eight repetitions of exercise #3: lat pull-down
One set of eight repetitions of exercise #4: hamstring curl
One set of eight repetitions of exercise #5: biceps curl
One set of eight repetitions of exercise #6: abdominal crunch
One set of eight repetitions of exercise #7: leg press
One set of eight repetitions of exercise #8: triceps cable press-down

Rest for sixty seconds between exercises, and rest for two or three minutes once you've completed the circuit. Then repeat the circuit. If you do a circuit like this one twice, it shouldn't take you much more than a half hour.

Traditionally, you do this type of training with machines, because you are moving pretty quickly from one exercise to another. If you choose to do this with free weights or bands, allow yourself a few extra seconds to go from one exercise to the next. There are two primary differences between your initial strength-training program and circuit training. One is that you don't perform multiple, consecutive sets of one exercise for a single muscle, but rather complete one full circuit—that is, one set of each exercise you plan to do that day. Rather than fatiguing the muscle, you will be focusing on moving quickly from one exercise to the next. This creates the other primary difference between your initial program of strength training and circuit training: Your rapid movement from one exercise to the next adds a significant cardiovascular component to your weight-training session.

A few tips for those of you who want to try circuit training:

- Look around the weight room at your gym. The machines may be situated in a circuit already, which makes it particularly easy for you to move from one station to the next.
- Don't be overly enthusiastic and try to complete more than two or three sets of each exercise. This type of training is more exhausting than you might at first realize.
- Paying attention to your form is still of paramount importance. Although you are moving quickly around the gym, you should not rush through each set.
- Be creative—if someone else is using a machine on your circuit, it's perfectly okay to substitute another exercise, either for a single circuit or for your entire workout session.
- Start with one or two circuit-training sessions a week, and don't do more than three in one week. Remember, you never want to exercise a specific muscle two days in a row, so you shouldn't circuit train more frequently than every other day.

2. *Try supersets.* The main advantage of this weight-training method is that you minimize the time you spend resting, both between sets and between different exercises. There are a couple of popular variations on this technique. In one, *instead of taking the usual minute or more rest period between sets,* you will complete all the sets of an exercise for

a specific muscle before moving on to an exercise for an opposing muscle. The first muscle you worked will recover while you're working its opposing muscle. For instance, after a set of biceps curls, pause briefly, no more than thirty seconds, and then do a set of triceps kick-backs.

When you first try this technique, perform only one set of each exercise. Focus on reducing your rest period between exercises, and pay attention to your form. After a week or two, you can add a second set immediately after the first. So in our example above, you'd do a set of biceps curls, pause briefly, then do a second set of the same exercise. You will just have completed a superset.

Another variation to working one muscle and then its opposing muscle is to do an exercise that works a large group of muscles, and then choose a second exercise that works just one of the muscles from that group. For instance, you may choose to do a set of squats, and follow it by a set of hamstring curls. The first exercise will work the quads, hamstrings, and glutes; the second will really zero in on the hamstrings, which have been "prefatigued" by the squats.

Although this technique can really shorten the time it takes to complete your strength training exercises, it is an intense type of training and may leave your muscles a bit more fatigued. Consider trying supersets during a holiday period when you're crunched for time, or during the summer when you want to spend more time pursuing outdoor activities.

3. *Try the pyramid system.* With this system, you perform multiple sets of an exercise, adding weight and reducing repetitions until you reach a peak (the top of the pyramid), and then move back down the pyramid by reducing weights and increasing repetitions until you are back where you started. Many weight lifters do five sets when they are using this

technique, but I recommend you start with just three sets. So, for example, your pyramid for biceps curls may look like this:

Set #1: twelve repetitions at five pounds
Set #2: eight or ten repetitions at ten pounds
Set #3: twelve repetitions at five pounds

There is also a technique called the modified pyramid, which is very popular among many exercisers. If you exercise in a gym, I'm sure you've seen people using this technique, although you may not have known what it was. In this system, you also add weight and decrease repetitions until you reach a peak—and then you stop, and move on to your next exercise. So for our biceps curl example, your modified pyramid could look like this:

Set #1: twelve repetitions at five pounds
Set #2: ten repetitions at eight pounds
Set #3: eight repetitions at ten pounds

4. *Try periodization. Periodization* is a type of weight training that is very useful if you are training for an event, or for a season of competition in any sport. It was initially developed and used by competitive weight lifters, but it's now popular with athletes in a variety of sports. The concept of periodization is based on the theory that muscle goes through three stages when it's introduced to weight training. According to this theory, the muscle's first response is shock (You want *me* to do *what?*). After several weight-training sessions, however, the muscle adapts to your demands. It gets stronger, responds more quickly, and masters the weight-training exercises. But once the challenge is conquered, the muscle gets bored and stops learning. Your muscles stop getting stronger, quicker. Imagine that this third stage coincides with an event you've been training for, or the begin-

ning of your sport's competitive season! Rather than capitalizing on your hard work, you'll put in a performance that's just ho-hum.

Periodization is a technique adopted by athletes to prevent this from happening. To try periodization, you'll need to sit down with a calendar and map out a training schedule. In the first few weeks, you'll plan to weight train several days a week, doing a higher number of repetitions using a smaller weight. Over the next few weeks, you'll gradually increase the amount of weight, but decrease the number of repetitions. After a few weeks, your muscles will be primed, and at their peak. Ideally, you should be at this stage a few weeks before your event or sports season begins. Now you can take advantage of your well-trained muscles and begin refining your sports-specific skills. For example, a runner might begin concentrating on speed workouts, and a soccer player might focus on agility drills.

Many athletes stop weight training once their competitive season begins, but a better technique is to continue some weight training to maintain strength. The experts'

How do I know which weight-lifting method is best for me? Each method has its own benefits. The best training method for you is the one you'll stick with. So experiment! Try circuit training if you want to maximize the aerobic benefit of weight training, or priority training if you want to emphasize strength. You may see the best results if you mix it up: for instance, try using bands for a few sessions, then alternate with circuit training using machines at the gym or priority training with free weights. Make your own rules!

opinions of the optimal amount of strength training for the maintenance stage varies, but a good rule of thumb is to perform only two or three exercises that target the muscles most important in your sport. Weight training during this stage is generally best done just two or three days a week, and it shouldn't take more than thirty minutes (sixty minutes for highly competitive elite athletes).

ALTERNATE METHODS OF STRENGTH TRAINING

Although traditionally strength training is often thought to be synonymous with weight training, strength training can be achieved in a variety of ways. Using the body's own weight, often referred to as resistance training, can be a very effective form of strength training. Several such methods that are currently popular include Pilates, Lotte Berk, and some types of yoga such as ashtanga. An advantage offered by these methods is that they emphasize the core muscles of the back and abdomen, which many women tend to neglect in other strength-training techniques.

Pilates

Named after its founder, Joseph Pilates, Pilates training uses the body's own resistance to improve strength and muscle tone. It combines moves from dance and gymnastics with yoga and strength training. Pilates developed this style of training to aid his own severe asthma and maximize his health. Today, Pilates-based exercise programs are styled after his focus on controlled breathing and strengthening of the body's core muscles in the abdomen and back. Originally practiced almost exclusively by dancers, Pilates-styled exercises can now be found in a variety of videotapes and exercise classes, as well as the basis for some injured athletes' rehabilitation programs. (Check the Resources at the end of this book for more information.)

Lotte Berk Method

Similar to Pilates, the Lotte Berk Method, named after the modern dancer whose career was cut short by a back injury, also combines strength and flexibility exercises into one workout. It incorporates a mix of modern and ballet dance moves with yoga and physical therapy exercises. Originally only in New York City, Lotte Berk moves can also be found in many suburban dance studios and aerobics classes.

Part Five of My Personal Exercise Program

Advancing Weight Training
Results of my first fitness assessment:

Results of my second fitness assessment:

Health goals I feel I'm meeting, or continuing to work toward:

To progress from this point, I'm going to try:

To help stay motivated, I will:

SAMPLE PROGRAM FOR PROGRESSION OF WEIGHT TRAINING

Paula, a forty-seven-year-old preschool teacher, began exercising four months ago to improve her daily stamina. For strength training, she used two videotapes, which included exercises using body weight for resistance (like modified push-ups), as well as small dumbbells. Paula progressed from two-pound dumbbells to five-pound ones. She now found it much easier to lift children, scramble from her knees to her feet, and end the day with enough energy to take her collie for a long walk. Her fifty-four-year-old sister was just diagnosed with osteoporosis, and Paula wanted to progress her own strength-training program with osteoporosis prevention in mind.

Results of first fitness assessment: Paula did four single leg squats, eleven crunches, and three modified push-ups.

Results of second fitness assessment: After four months, Paula easily did ten single leg squats, twenty crunches, and twelve modified push-ups.

The *health benefits* Paula credited to exercise were more energy and stamina, a drop in dress size, stress reduction, better sleep, and enhanced general health. Her new goal was to maximize her weight training for osteoporosis prevention.

To progress, she began using the modified pyramid training technique. Instead of staying with three sets of ten repetitions with a five-pound weight, she performed the following:

Set #1: twelve repetitions at five pounds
Set #2: ten repetitions at six pounds
Set #3: eight repetitions at eight pounds

She also bought a videotape of tai chi, and she began balance training.

To help stay motivated, Paula made a weekly date with her sister to take a local tai chi class together. She splurged on several new sleeveless blouses to showcase her toned shoulders and arms.

CHAPTER 7

CONQUERING NEW
FITNESS CHALLENGES

EVERY DAY, at least one woman actually *apologizes* for coming to see me at the Women's Sports Medicine Center. When I walk in the door, she'll meet my eyes and hesitantly say something like "I should tell you right away, I'm not an athlete." Then she goes on to tell me about whatever problem brought her to our center, like the knee pain she developed running or the sore shoulder she's gotten weight training. She's usually amazed (and then thrilled!) when I tell her that in my view, she *is* an athlete. Maybe not a competitive one, usually not a professional one, but she's still an athlete. And any woman, whether or not she thinks of herself as an athlete, can train for an event.

TRAINING FOR AN EVENT:
NOT FOR "ATHLETES" ONLY

Over the past decade, I have met many "ordinary" women who compete in triathlons, run marathons, climb some of the world's highest peaks, swim across huge bodies of water, and cycle vast distances. These women are ordinary in the sense that they are not professional athletes. They are schoolteachers, pharmacists, students, writers, homemakers, attorneys, nurses, accountants, secretaries. They are mothers, daughters, sisters. They are often more surprised than anyone else when they acknowledge their desire to train for and complete such a feat of physical fitness. And many times, a woman has told me that what began as a dream changed her life.

Andrea, for instance. A twenty-nine-year-old overweight single mother of two, she began a walking program, got talked into walking in a 10-kilometer race (6.2 miles) to benefit breast cancer research, and ultimately completed the women-only Danskin triathalon. Or Jodi, a forty-three-year-old, depressed, recently divorced veterinarian who entered and completed the New York City Marathon. And Carol, a thirty-six-year-old chain-smoking paralegal whose firm's work on behalf of a disabled athlete rekindled her childhood interest in swimming. She stopped smoking, then trained for and ultimately completed a 2-mile open-water swim.

While intense training changed these women's bodies, each of them said that it was the effect on her mind that made the biggest difference in her life. What started as a dream, a fantasy, became real, and made them each realize that achievement in other areas was only a dream away.

Eventually, Carol went to law school. Jodi said that competing gave her the self-confidence to date again. And Andrea overcame the intimidation of relocating to accept a promising job offer.

TRAINING FOR AN EVENT IS A GREAT MOTIVATOR

Some studies have shown that women who have the vague goal of getting in shape have a hard time committing to an exercise program, but that those who have a more concrete challenge in mind succeed at making exercise an important part of their lives. *This is one of the reasons I think it's so important for you to set your own health goals to work toward.* If attaining the health goals you've already established isn't enough to keep you sticking to the exercise program you designed, consider training for a specific event. The event you choose could be anything from a family bicycling vacation to the Ironman Triathlon. There are literally thousands of organized events you can choose from, including fun runs, 5K or 10K (3.1 or 6.2 miles, respectively) walks and runs, bike rides, rowing and swimming competitions, inline skating events, biathlons (two events, like running and bicycling, rolled into one) or triathlons (usually swimming, bicycling, and running), and marathons. Many of these benefit charities, local civic organizations, and health research. A little sleuthing in local newspapers, nonprofit organizations, the chamber of commerce, websites, or fitness magazines will help you to choose among the many options. The Resources at the back of this book have several suggestions for help finding events.

Many women find that training for such an event makes it easier to stay committed to an exercise program. If you join them, you'll find that daily tasks don't distract you the same way they did when your exercise was less focused. And along the way to the event you're training for, a wonderful thing will happen. Perhaps without your realizing it, your commitment to exercise will establish permanent residence in your lifestyle.

Do *you* have a hidden fitness fantasy?

ESTABLISHING A TRAINING PLAN

Once you've decided to train for an event, it's critical that you develop a sound plan that will get you to the finish line healthy and injury-free. Like your original exercise program, your event training schedule needs to be individualized. *This is especially important if you are new to the type of event in which you'll be participating.* For instance, even if you've been jogging a few days each week, training for a marathon will require more than just increasing your mileage. You'll need to learn different training techniques, such as the importance of doing speed work, hill runs, and distance runs. There are many resources available to help you plan a training program, but remember, they are just general guidelines. Only *you* can factor in the personal information that will make your training program truly successful.

Ironically, I've often found that the women who don't consider themselves athletes are much better at developing and sticking with a personalized training program. Don't make the mistake of assuming that a friend or spouse who has been performing a particular activity is automatically an expert. Unless a friend or spouse is a professional who teaches the activity for a living, don't rely on his or her experience to guide you. Plan to use him or her for adjunct advice, not as your coach. Use the following tips to design a smart, individualized training program.

Tips for Training for an Event

1. *Do your homework.* Learning about training for an event in advance of actually beginning the training process will give you a realistic idea of (a) how much time it takes to train for the event you've chosen, (b) what the components of training should be, (c) what equipment, including appropriate shoes, you'll need. Be sure the scheduled date for the event is far enough away to leave you ample time to train appropriately.

2. *Establish a base* of comfort and competence with the particular activity involved before you begin training. For instance, if you want to train for a marathon, you should already be running a minimum of 15 miles a week before you begin a training schedule.

3. *Follow the 10 percent rule.* Increase the time or distance of your activity by no more than 10 to 15 percent each week. Using the marathon example, if you're currently running 20 total miles in a week, progress to running 22 total miles, then 25, and so on. *One of the most common causes of injury is ignorance of this basic rule.*

4. *Take rest days.* Days of rest, in which you do not train, are critical to avoid injury and prevent overtraining. I recommend that novices rest two days each week; more experienced athletes may need only one rest day each week.

5. *Change one thing at a time.* Don't begin all the different training strategies in the same week. If you're trying your first hill run this week, wait until next week for your first trial of speed work.

6. *Don't try to make up for missed training sessions.* Unexpected interruptions are a part of life. Pick up where you left off, and don't worry about what you missed. If you had a cold or other illness and missed a few days, go back to your last easy workout and repeat that. Make sure you feel healthy and energetic before you progress your training.

7. *Cross-train.* Consider an alternate activity once a week, especially if your primary activity is an impact one. Riding a bike, swimming, or running in a pool will give you a great cardiovascular workout while resting your bones and joints from the demands of impact.

8. *Don't ignore pain.* Some muscle soreness is not unexpected, but pain is a signal that something is wrong. Ignoring pain is a sure ticket to making an injury worse.

9. *If you train with a partner, make sure you're roughly equals.* Training with a partner or group at least one day a week is great for motivation and camaradarie, and will inspire you to push yourself. But if a training partner is consistently ahead of you, you're likely to become discouraged and think of quitting. Worse, you risk injury. If you're consistently ahead of your partner, you will get frustrated that you're being held back, and will lose the benefit of having someone push you to improve.

10. *Keep a training log.* Not only does writing it down help you keep track of your planned training schedule, it's also a great record of your personal progress. Pull it out on days when you're feeling down about anything, and it will re-

mind you of your ability to work hard to conquer challenges. Keep a record of your body's response to training, such as training heart rate and muscle soreness. It's also a good idea to chart your resting heart rate. Resting heart rate is your heart rate when you are lying or sitting still, and it's a good measure of underlying fitness. The more fit you are, the lower your resting heart rate will be. Very fit athletes often have a resting heart rate in the forties or fifties. Increases in your resting heart rate are often a warning sign that you are training excessively and need to build in more rest days.

11. *Pay attention to diet and fluid intake.* The difference between success and failure, injury and health, strength and weakness may be as simple as what you put (or don't put) in your mouth. (See chapter 9 on eating like an athlete.)

12. *Be flexible.* The training process should be fun and exciting, not another chore to add to your to-do list. If, on occasion, you can't fit your planned workout into your day, just do a shorter one. Remember, anything is better than nothing. Don't lose sight of the fact that every minute you spend in activity is an investment in your *health.*

OVERTRAINING: LEARNING THE VALUE OF QUALITY, NOT QUANTITY

I often give community lectures about the health benefits of exercise. After one such lecture to employees of a large corporation, I got a phone call from Susan, the woman who had arranged the session, telling me that she had never realized how important exercise was, and that she was making a personal commitment to exercise to lower her blood pressure and manage her weight. She began a walking program, progressed to running, and eventually to racing. Susan achieved her health goals and began pushing herself to achieve more. Unfortunately, she also became my patient. Susan was so enthusiastic about exercise and competing that she pushed herself too hard, too fast. As a result, she developed several injuries caused by *overtraining.*

Simply put, overtraining is an imbalance between training and recovery. Elite-level athletes of the seventies and eighties learned the hard way that too much training leads to injuries and poor performance. Today, athletes and their coaches have turned their attention to quality rather than quantity workouts. But as the popularity of competitions like the marathon has skyrocketed, more and more recreational athletes have begun making the mistakes characteristic of overtraining.

Some women don't seem to realize that when it comes to exercise, you *can* get too much of a good thing. Excessive amounts of exercise can have many detrimental effects. Obviously, it increases your risk of injury, but it can also have more subtle—and possibly more important—effects on your health. For instance, while moderate amounts of exercise stimulate the immune system, overtraining can actually suppress the immune system. Researchers don't yet understand why this happens, but they have documented lower amounts of disease-fighting cells in the circulation of overtrained athletes. We also know that after strenuous events like a marathon, many runners are especially vulnerable to viral infections. I recommend that women who participate in a very challenging event like a marathon be especially vigilant about avoiding close contact with ill friends and family for a few days thereafter.

Recognizing the Signs of Overtraining

How do you know if your zeal to train for an event is overriding your body's need for rest? Check your resting heart rate first thing in the morning for several days. If, on average, it's higher than your training log shows it was previously, chances are you are overtraining. Be honest in assessing yourself for the warning signs of overtraining, like injury, fatigue, and disappointing performance. Too many athletes think poor performance means they aren't training hard enough, when in reality they are overtraining. Then take a close look at your life outside of training to make sure you're not missing any of the other telltale signs. And finally, ask your doctor to evaluate you for other common causes of fatigue, like anemia. I will never forget Terry, a hard-driving collegiate volleyball player, whose coach made her sit out a

---

WARNING SIGNALS OF OVERTRAINING

- Pain or progressive discomfort, during or after exercise
- Fatigue that frequently limits your workout
- Loss of interest in your training
- Declining performance
- "Heavy" legs, or muscle soreness affecting your training

And examine your life outside of training for:

- Disturbed sleep
- Feeling blue
- Diminished sex drive
- Frequent infections, including colds
- Weight loss

---

week for overtraining. When her fatigue worsened despite the rest, she came to see me for a medical evaluation. Her fatigue turned out to be caused by pregnancy!

MASTERING A NEW SPORT

During the spring of 2001, as I watched the inaugural game of the newly created Women's United Soccer Association, I was struck by two thoughts simultaneously. The first was that the women I was watching race around the field were strong, fast, and agile: in other words, impressively fit. The second was that they were having a great time playing their game.

It isn't just a coincidence that all our efforts to get fit are described as "*working* out," but when it comes to sports, we say we're "*playing.*" The ability to play and enjoy a sport is a wonderful reward for all the hard work it takes to achieve a solid foundation of fitness. But if you skipped ahead to this chapter of the book, go back to the beginning: it's imperative that total fitness comes first! As one of my colleagues, Dr. Mark Sherman, is fond of saying, "Don't play your sport to get into shape . . . get into shape to play your sport." Becoming fit first will help you master a new sport and improve your athletic performance, and it will provide insurance against many athletic injuries.

Perhaps even more important for women, becoming fit helps develop physical confidence, which is crucial to mastering a new sport. In my experience, men are generally not intimidated by learning a new sport, but women often are. I believe this is largely because women often underestimate themselves, lacking confidence that they can rise to the physical challenges of a new sport. But when women become fit first, they develop a wonderful appreciation for their bodies' physical capabilities, and sports are no longer intimidating—just fun.

DEVELOPING SPORTS-SPECIFIC SKILLS

Toni exercised with aerobics tapes at home a few days a week. When her husband asked her to join his co-ed softball team, she was flattered. She was also apprehensive, because she wasn't sure if she was in good enough shape to join the team.

Toni didn't have to worry about her level of physical conditioning: from her aerobics tapes she had developed a moderate level of fitness, which was adequate to begin playing softball. But she did need to take two steps before hitting the softball diamond. First, she needed to learn the game's rules and lingo, which she could easily master with a little help from her husband. Just having a basic knowledge of the rules and terms her teammates would use to communicate gave her a crucial first dose of confidence. Second, she needed to practice holding and swinging a bat; hitting, catching, and throwing a ball; and sprinting. In other words, she needed to develop sports-specific skills.

You may think that because you're physically fit you'll be a natural at your newly chosen sport. Athletes will tell you differently. Although some athletes may have a special aptitude for a certain sport, most of them feel that their athletic competence is a combination of talent and hard work. When I was hosting *Recipe for Health,* a "healthy lifestyles" television show on Food Network, I had an opportunity to interview some terrific female athletes, including WNBA star

Theresa Weatherspoon and Olympic gold medal–winning gymnast Kerri Strug. These and other top athletes confirmed over and over, no matter how fit you are, or how athletic you've been, *practice, practice, and more practice* is what it takes to conquer a new sport.

Failure to realize that playing different sports requires practicing different skills is one of the most common mistakes made by recreational athletes. For example, one of my patients, Carla, developed a solid fitness base through running 15 miles each week. She took a few tennis lessons while on a recent vacation and was amazed to find she couldn't get to the ball quickly enough on the tennis court. Carla jumped to the conclusion that she was no good at tennis. In reality, it was simply that she hadn't learned the skills necessary to play tennis. Although she was proficient at running straight ahead at a low to moderate intensity, her body hadn't been trained to make the quick, stop-and-go type movements needed for tennis. Nor had she developed the necessary hand-eye coordination or upper-extremity muscle strength and endurance. Carla simply needed to acquire and practice the skills that are specific to tennis.

While sports-specific skills are important for all athletes to learn, I have found that women particularly benefit from this type of training, largely because of the confidence it instills. Novice female athletes, especially those over thirty, frequently feel intimidated by others' athletic abilities and are apologetic for their own perceived shortcomings. Practicing sports-specific skills is a great way to break a new sport into smaller, more easily mastered segments. Conquering even one specific drill, such as learning to serve a tennis ball, catch a softball, or drive a golf ball, can make an inexperienced athlete feel more confident in her new sport.

Once you realize the importance of learning sports-specific skills, it's generally easy to find someone to introduce you to a few skill-enhancing drills. Most athletes are so enthusiastic about their favorite sports that they're more

PLYOMETRICS

Plyometrics are exercises that top-level athletes rely on to develop explosive power. Also known as *jump training,* plyometrics have been used for years by track and field athletes, football and basketball players, and tennis stars. It's the secret to a higher vertical jump; fast, agile feet; and the ability to jump the net at the end of the tennis match. In the past decade, this type of training has become much more popular among personal trainers and the general public. *While very effective, it is a technique for advanced exercisers and athletes only.* One of the worst injuries I've ever seen sustained in the gym occurred when a personal trainer pushed a woman with a low level of fitness to try a plyometric drill involving jumping quickly and repetitively over a step. She fatigued rapidly, stumbled, and fractured two bones in her ankle.

If you have a moderate to high level of fitness, plyometrics may be just what the doctor ordered to give you a burst of power for jumping and sprinting. If you want to give it a try, start with fifteen to twenty minutes of jump-training drills done after a brief warm-up but before the rest of your workout. (If your muscles are already fatigued, you're much more likely to suffer an injury.) Because this method of training is so intense, I don't recommend you try it more than once a week. You can find illustrated instructions in a variety of sources, or you can start with three moves you practiced as a child: hopscotch, leapfrog, and jumping rope. Exaggerate those movements, and you'll be on your way to becoming a plyometrics fan.

than happy to teach you the basics. You can also learn from coaches and private instructors. And be sure that you ask them to teach you a few techniques that you can practice when you're alone.

CHOOSING A NEW SPORT

Even if you've never played a sport—any sport—before, don't let that stop you now. There are more athletic opportunities available to girls and women of all ages than ever before. But just as your personal fitness program needed to be customized, so does your foray into the wonderful world of sports. To start, ask yourself the following questions:

Do I Have a Personal Preference for a Team vs. an Individual Sport?

Some women are drawn to team sports like softball, volleyball, and soccer, where participation requires group effort. They like the social contacts as well as the opportunity to compete and win. Others enjoy competing, but prefer an independently performed activity, like tennis or bike racing. If you prefer the latter, consider joining a "club sport," which allows you to pursue an individual sport while reaping the rewards of teamwork.

Clubs for participants in many sports, like running, bicycling, rowing, and swimming offer the fitness enthusiasts a chance to join a team despite the fact that their sport is not a traditional team sport. Such clubs are very popular among many of my patients, and they offer countless benefits beyond the obvious social ones. Joining a group whose members enjoy the same sport provides instant camaraderie and motivation, and is one of the best ways to break through fitness plateaus. Competition, whether against your own personal best or against your teammates, can be friendly and low-key, but can still ultimately improve your athletic performance. Other pluses of team training include exposure to experienced coaches, enough variety to keep workouts interesting, encouragement, and companionship.

Do I Have Any Particular Physical Strengths or Weaknesses That Might Affect My Performance in Certain Sports?

This is your opportunity to play to your strengths! For instance, a woman who easily developed strong back and shoulder muscles through her weight training program may gravitate toward a swim club, whereas a woman with particularly strong legs may want to try mountain biking. A runner who finds speed is not her strong suit might try distance running or another sport that emphasizes endurance, rather than one that requires faster sprinting.

Do I Have Any Health Concerns That Might Affect My Choice of Sports?

While it's important to take your personal health into account, having a chronic illness doesn't mean you can't play sports. Asthma, for example, affects a tremendous number of sports participants, including many gold medal–winning Olympic athletes! Talk to your doctor about whether or not any illness you have or medication you take should influence your choice of sports. For instance, a woman who's had a difficult-to-control seizure disorder should choose a sport other than swimming, because having a seizure while in the water would place her at unacceptable risk of drowning. However, a woman with asthma may do best with swimming, because the wetness of the environment is friendlier to asthmatic lungs than a drier environment is. A woman who has vision difficulties subsequent to eye disease or eye surgery should choose a sport in which hand-eye coordination is not critically important, whereas one with osteoporosis should avoid activities with higher risks of falls, and so on.

Are There Financial or Geographic Factors I Need to Consider?

This is simply a matter of practicality. Golf, for instance, is an expensive sport that requires a significant commitment of both time and financial resources, as well as available courses for play. Basketball, on the other hand, can be played in numerous environs and requires only access to a court, proper shoes, and a ball. For city dwellers, finding space to pursue your choice of sports can be one of its biggest challenges, whereas those in rural areas might have access to facilities but more trouble finding enough players to create a team.

CHOOSING THE RIGHT GEAR FOR YOUR CHOSEN SPORT

It's easy to find out what gear you need for a particular sport; the harder part is finding the gear that's right for *you*. Whether or not you and your gear are a match made in heaven can have a profound effect on the success of your new endeavor. Until the past few years, women had to make do with gear designed for men. In general, women are shorter and lighter than men, have a lower center of gravity, and have increased angles at the knees and elbows. Because of these and other physical differences, gear designed for a man is frequently a poor fit for a woman. For years, improperly fitting gear has been a cause of frustration for female athletes and has been blamed for everything from poor performances to injuries.

Today, however, smart female athletes don't settle for a poor fit. Sporting goods companies recognize that not only are women becoming more active, they have real buying power. For instance, in the last few years, women have actually outspent men on athletic shoes, causing the sports marketing world to take notice. Unfortunately, some companies seem to think that catering to female athletes simply means scaling down the size of a product and painting it pink. Thankfully, other companies take women athletes more seriously and have begun to create products specifically designed for women. For instance, awareness of the difference in hand size between elite male and female basketball players led the women's professional basketball league, the WNBA, to design a ball smaller than the one used in the men's league, the NBA. And until recently, companies that made soccer cleats made only adult and child models; thanks to the tremendous explosion of interest in women's soccer, companies are beginning to make cleats sized and shaped for a woman's foot.

So how do you get the gear that's the right fit for you? Become an educated consumer. Be aware that most gear traditionally *was* designed for men, so don't be afraid to ask questions about equipment you are interested in purchasing, renting, or using at the gym. Find out exactly which features influence the way a piece of equipment fits. Search out companies with experience in making gear and apparel for professional and collegiate women athletes. If your local sporting goods store doesn't already carry gear designed specifically for women, ask them to start stocking it.

Other Tips for Choosing the Right Equipment

For racket sports: Pay attention to the size of the grip. Place the racket in your palm and wrap your fingers around it. If there is a gap of more than one-half to three-quarters of an inch between your fingertips and palm, it's probably too big. Also, because women tend to have more upper body weakness than men, they may prefer a somewhat stiffer racket. This is especially true of beginners.

For bicycles: Some women like the mixte style frame (the original "women's bike"), but many prefer the sturdier design of the "diamond" frame ("men's bike"). The *shape* of the frame is purely a matter of choice; the *size* of the frame is what's critical in preventing the back, shoulder, and neck pain that women frequently develop riding these bikes. This is because women usually need a bike with a shorter reach to the handlebars (determined by the length of the top tube) than men's bikes traditionally have. Look for a bicycle with features geared to women, such as a shorter top tube made for a women's frame, shorter brake levers, and a wider seat. Make sure you have enough clearance from your crotch to the top tube (at least an inch on a road bike, at least twice that for a mountain bike). Your reach to the handlebars should allow your arms to feel relaxed while your elbows remain bent. And consider a saddle designed specifically for the female anatomy, or one that's gel-padded, for a more comfortable ride. Remember that wearing padded shorts and gloves for biking is not just a comfort factor, it can help protect nerves in the pelvic area and wrist from pressure.

There are a few companies, such as Terry, whose primary focus is bikes built specifically for women; others, including Cannondale, make a few models geared toward women. Trek has an entire line designated WSD, or Women's Specific Design. Still others make only unisex bicycles, but

CHOOSING A SPORTS BRA

Until the last decade, women were stuck with one basic style of sports bra, the pull-over-the-head model. Fast-forward to the twenty-first century, and you have your choice of an unending variety of underwire, zip-front, hook-in-back, wide-strapped, and T-back models. How's a girl to choose?

It's pretty simple, once you get past the advertising, zippy colors, and mental photo of Brandi Chastain whipping off her jersey after the 1999 Women's World Cup Soccer finals. Despite all the hoopla, there are really just two basic models: the compression bra, which is the classic pull-over-your-head style; and the encapsulation bra, which is styled with two separate cups just like the standard daily-wear bra. The former is often preferred by smaller-breasted women (A and B cups), while the encapsulation style is more comfortable for larger-breasted women. Try both styles and see what works for you. Whichever style you choose, the bra should be supportive from above (provided by wide, solid straps with minimal vertical stretch) and from below (provided by a flat rib band or underwire). Look for models that minimize breast motion, and avoid seams across nipples. Try moving in ways that mimic your sport or fitness activity (for instance, jog in place) to be sure the bra stays put and is comfortable.

have a wider selection of frame and component sizes, so they can be custom-fit to a woman's unique form.

For other equipment, from bats to golf clubs: Look for lighter, shorter versions of traditional men's gear. Ask a professional to size you. It's worth it, because your height, stance, and swing all influence what's best for you and your game. And remember to get appropriate safety equipment, such as goggles and helmets.

A final note: If you know what you need, but not where to find it, check out one of the growing number of athletic-gear companies that cater to women, such as Title 9 Sports, The Female Athlete, or Athleta. Consult the Resources in the back of this book for more information.

PART 4

WHAT EVERY ACTIVE WOMAN NEEDS TO KNOW ABOUT NUTRITION

CHAPTER 8

EXERCISE AND WEIGHT LOSS

ON ANY GIVEN DAY, thousands of women are starting—or quitting—diet or exercise programs for weight control. In my practice, some of the questions I am most frequently asked revolve around exercise for weight loss. The tremendous number of revolutionary diet programs, cookbooks, magazine articles, and videos that appear each year suggests that weight loss is like the Holy Grail: sought by many but achieved by few. It seems that every day one of my patients brings in an advertisement for the latest weapon in the war against excess body fat, hoping that I will be as enthusiastic as the testimonials produced by the product's company. And they never fail to be disappointed when I tell them the truth: It won't work. *There is no dietary gimmick, nutritional supplement, or special exercise that is the universal key to successful weight loss.* To lose weight (and keep it off) simply requires you to understand and respond to your own body's unique energy needs. In a nutshell, this means figuring out how to balance your energy intake (in the form of food) with your energy output.

CALCULATING YOUR OWN ENERGY OUTPUT

Sally, a forty-four-year-old overweight pharmacist, was frustrated that, despite trying every diet, exercise, and weight-loss aid, she had been unable to achieve lasting weight loss. She was ready to give up, saying she had been "cursed with a slow metabolism."

The concept of *metabolism* refers to a complex interaction between a number of chemical reactions, which all work together to keep the body functioning normally. Even if you spend the whole day just lying in bed, your metabolism keeps working to regulate your body temperature, mend and replace damaged tissue, send hormones out into circulation, and allow your brain to process signals from the rest of your body. Your liver and kidneys continue to remove waste products from the bloodstream, and your heart continues to beat at a constant pace. All of these processes require a basic amount of energy, referred to as the *resting metabolic rate (RMR).*

Many patients are surprised when I explain to them how much energy—in the form of calories—the resting metabolic rate represents. Although it varies from individual to individual, just to keep your body alive and performing these basic functions requires approximately 10 calories per pound of body weight. So, for instance, a 150-pound woman like Sally has an estimated RMR requiring 1,500 calories a day.

It is important to realize that this estimated metabolic rate can be influenced by a wide variety of factors, and can even vary from day to day. For instance, having a fever temporarily increases the metabolic rate, which is one reason many people notice a slight weight loss after an illness. On the other hand, significantly restricting calories through dieting triggers a complex chain of events in the body, resulting in a *decrease* in the metabolic rate. This process probably was a tremendous benefit in the distant past, when food sources were sometimes scarce. By slowing down its basic requirements, the human body could survive until more food was available. However, the fact that there is such a slowdown in the metabolic rate when there is such a significant drop in calorie intake ironically sabotages low-calorie diets.

The resting metabolic rate represents the body's *minimum* energy requirements, and it's usually two-thirds to three-quarters of the total daily energy needs. It can be estimated by:

$$RMR = \text{weight in pounds} \times 10$$

The rest of the daily energy requirement is determined by the amount of usual physical activity any individual does in a day. This can be estimated by the following generalities:

If you are sedentary, additional energy required is approximately 30 percent of RMR.

If you are somewhat active, additional energy required is approximately 40 percent of RMR.

If you are moderately active, additional energy required is approximately 50 percent of RMR.

If you are very active, additional energy required is approximately 75 percent of RMR.

If you are extremely active, additional energy required is approximately 100 percent of RMR.

If you perform vigorous exercise, you will require even more calories; exactly how many depends on your size, exercise choice, duration, and intensity.

Let's use Sally as an example. Sally described herself as sedentary, because she drives to her job as a pharmacist, sits on a stool behind the counter for most of the day, then drives home and spends most of the evening sitting on the couch watching television. We estimated her total daily energy output as:

RMR = 150 (Sally's weight) × 10 = 1500
Additional energy required = 30 percent × 1500 = 450
Total energy required = 1,950 calories per day

And on days when Sally is more active, whether from chores like washing dishes and mowing the lawn or by tossing a Frisbee with her son at the beach, her calorie needs are even higher. Sally was flabbergasted. How could that possibly be anywhere close to the number of calories she needed in a day, she asked, when she had trouble losing weight on a 1,200-calorie-a-day diet? The answer: Cutting back to 1,200 calories a day triggered a warning signal for her body to lower its metabolic rate. It also left Sally feeling hungry, tired, and miserable, which in turn sabotaged her intention to exercise. On those occasions when she was able to lose weight, she lost muscle as well as fat. Losing muscle meant losing some of the most metabolically active tissue in her body (see page 14), which decreased her metabolic rate even further. She felt sluggish and deprived, and started thinking about ice cream and cookies several times each day. Pretty soon, she was at the ice cream shop next door to the pharmacy, eating a double banana split with extra chocolate sauce. Upset with herself for blowing the diet, she was back at the ice cream shop the next day, assuaging her feelings of guilt and self-loathing with more ice cream.

To achieve lasting weight loss, Sally simply needed to reduce her calorie intake less drastically and keep her commitment to exercise. Decreasing her calorie intake by just 10 to 20 percent (roughly 200 to 400 calories) would allow her to eat enough to keep her energy up, prevent that feeling of deprivation that previously triggered her ice cream binge, and keep her metabolic rate from plummeting. And exercise would help her to lose weight and keep it off.

ESTIMATE YOUR OWN DAILY CALORIE NEEDS

My RMR = _____ (my weight in pounds) × 10 calories per pound = __A__ calories

Additional calories based on level of daily activity = _____ percent × __A__ = __B__ additional calories

A + B = __C__

C = estimate of my own energy output

If your goal is weight loss, plan to eat 10 to 20 percent fewer calories than this estimate, and don't forget to exercise! (Remember that the extra calories you burn through exercise are not factored into this estimate for your RMR.)

HOW EXERCISE HELPS YOU BURN CALORIES AND LOSE WEIGHT

Let's go back to the image of your body as a complex machine, such as a luxury sports car. If you want to go for a drive, you'll need to buy fuel, or units of energy, called gallons of gasoline. When you buy gasoline for the car, you can get just enough to cover your travel needs for the day, or you can fill the tank as "storage." If you fill the tank but then rarely use the car, all the excess fuel will remain in the tank, unused.

Calories are your body's gallons of gasoline: they are the units of energy that provide the fuel for your body to function. Whatever you're doing—reading the words on this page, tying a shoe, lifting a child, running, even eating or sleeping—is powered by calories. Like buying gasoline for your car, you can eat just enough calories to power you through your day, or you can eat extra ones and put them in a "storage tank." A small number of calories will be stored in the muscles, and the rest will be stored in your body's main storage tank: fat.

We all need some fat around: it cushions our internal organs, provides a good source of energy for prolonged activities, and helps insulate us from the cold. But many women are walking around with more fat stored than they're ever going to be able to use. These excess stores of fuel become a significant burden for the rest of your hardworking body. Even if you know you'll probably never need them, as long as you hang on to the extra calories, your body has to maintain their storage. That means your heart has to pump more nutrient-rich blood to sustain your fat stores; your joints strain under the extra bulk they must carry; even your skin has to stretch to cover the growing fat stores. And each day that you carry the excess fat increases your risk of life-threatening diseases like heart disease and diabetes.

But getting rid of the extra fat stores takes all that extra strain off the system, which suddenly leaves you with a lot more energy. Think about how you feel when you carry a heavy package or bag: When you finally set it down, you feel relieved. You can move more quickly and easily because you're no longer carrying a heavy burden. Your body has the same response when you shed unneeded pounds. And despite all the hoopla of popular diet plans, weight loss just boils down to a simple bit of math:

1 pound = 3,500 calories of energy

This is true for every single one of us, no matter what our size, gender, or ethnicity; no matter what our health, eating habits, exercise history, or metabolic rate. Therefore, to lose one pound of fat, you need to lose 3,500 calories. Considering that *every body function*—even breathing!—requires you to burn some calories, it's not that hard to start getting rid of some of the extra ones. When you exercise, many of your body's functions kick into high gear and burn more fuel (calories) in the process. And because exercise stimulates metabolism, you continue burning a few extra calories per hour for several hours after you stop exercising. And if you exercise by weight training, the extra muscle that you develop will constantly burn extra calories, even when you're fast asleep!

The exact number of calories burned during an exercise session is determined by a variety of factors. Many women forget that if they were not exercising, they would be burning some calories anyway, even if just while sitting on the couch watching television (remember RMR?). So if you want to try to estimate the calorie cost of any activity, you must estimate the *difference* between the number of calories you burned while doing that exercise and those that you would have used for your usual activity.

Three of the previously described fitness factors—which activity is chosen, how long it is done, and how intensely it is performed—affect how many calories are burned. Additionally, the weight of the individual exerciser affects the number of calories burned: The more you weigh, the more calories you'll actually use. Be aware that many of the tables that exist to allow exercisers to estimate their calorie expenditure are actually based on *men weighing an average of 150 pounds.* I find the tables that estimate calorie expenditure per minute per pound, and take intensity into account, are more reliable. But remember, the more muscle you have, the more calories you'll actually burn . . . and the less you have, the fewer you burn. So the smartest way to use calorie-expenditure charts is as an *estimate:* apply the general principles and then *individualize* them.

MUSCLE MATTERS

Every woman has noticed that men seem to have a much easier time when it comes to losing weight. This is largely because women have about 10 percent more body fat and up to 30 percent less muscle than men. Because muscle is more metabolically active than fat, women will generally have a resting metabolic rate (RMR) at least 5 to 10 percent lower than men, which many people refer to as a slower metabolism. Their higher rate of metabolism gives men an advantage in weight loss because it allows them to burn a minimum of 5 to 10 percent more calories each day. That's why weight training is so important for women who want to lose weight: more muscle translates into a higher RMR, for women as well as men.

Exercising women, take heart: There is one bright spot to having higher fat stores, in that some researchers now believe that the combination of lighter bones and relatively higher body fat may prove to be an advantage in ultra-endurance events, particularly swimming.

Activity	Effort	_____ Body Weight _____					
		100 lb	120 lb	140 lb	160 lb	180 lb	200 lb
Walking	2.5 MPH	2.4	2.9	3.3	3.8	4.3	4.8
	4.0 MPH	3.4	4.1	4.7	5.4	6.1	6.8
Running	5.0 MPH	6.4	7.6	8.9	10.2	11.5	12.7
	6.0 MPH	8.0	9.5	11.1	12.7	14.3	15.9
	8.0 MPH	10.7	12.9	15.0	17.2	19.3	21.5
Bicycling	10 MPH	4.0	4.8	5.6	6.4	7.2	8.0
	15 MPH	8.0	9.5	11.1	12.7	14.3	15.9
Aerobics	Low impact	4.0	4.8	5.6	6.4	7.2	8.0
	High impact	5.6	6.7	7.8	8.9	10.0	11.1
Swimming	Leisurely	4.8	5.7	6.7	7.6	8.6	9.5
	Lap swimming	7.6	9.1	10.6	12.1	13.6	15.1
Stair stepper	Level 4	4.8	5.7	6.7	7.6	8.6	9.5
	Level 8	7.6	9.1	10.6	12.1	13.6	15.1
Skiing downhill	Moderate	4.8	5.7	6.7	7.6	8.6	9.5
Skiing X country	Moderate	6.4	7.6	8.9	10.2	11.5	12.7
Hiking	3 MPH	4.5	5.4	6.3	7.3	8.2	9.1

Estimated calories burned per minute by activity and body weight.
Actual calories burned may vary depending on effort, level of fitness, and environmental conditions.

One additional caveat: Although there are always 3,500 calories of energy generated from a pound of fat, your body prefers to stay in a set weight range. We don't know all the factors that determine this range, but genetics certainly plays a role. The upside of having a set weight is that if you overeat a bit, your body can increase its usual metabolic pace to get rid of a few extra calories. However, if your weight drops below the set weight it is accustomed to, you may burn fewer calories. *That doesn't mean you will not be able to lose the extra pounds,* it just means you may lose it more slowly than you anticipated.

WHY EXERCISE ALONE IS NOT ENOUGH

Carrie's large family had frequent cookouts and birthday parties, complete with lots of chips, sodas, and desserts. When Carrie realized that she was gaining weight with each passing celebration, she decided to begin an exercise program to lose the extra pounds.

When Carrie came to talk to me about starting an exercise program, her goal was simple: She planned to lose weight through exercise so that she could continue to enjoy her family's frequent calorie-laden celebrations without worrying about her weight. Since the family typically got together twice a month, Carrie figured that exercising twice a week should more than take care of the extra calories. Unfortunately, the math didn't work in Carrie's favor. While starting an exercise program would certainly help her burn off some of the extra calories, her plan wasn't likely to result in the weight loss she anticipated. Between chips, sodas, burgers, and her favorite gooey deserts, Carrie was eating almost

5,000 calories at each family gathering. That translated into 10,000 extra calories a month! Since Carrie was interested in a walking program twice a week, or eight days each month, she would have to burn over 1,200 additional calories in each exercise session to compensate for the extra calories.

Carrie was making two very common mistakes: She was underestimating the number of calories she was consuming at the family gatherings, and she was overestimating the impact of exercise on weight loss. To achieve her goal, Carrie needed to trim some of the excess calories from her weekend celebrations, and at the same time increase her caloric expenditure through exercise.

Additionally, she had never given any thought to the nutritional content of the high-fat foods she was consuming. When I mentioned that she was consuming lots of fat and sugar at these cookouts, Carrie's response was that if she began exercising and paid attention to *how much* she was eating, *what* she ate wouldn't matter. Like many women, Carrie assumed that exercise eliminates the need to monitor dietary content. This is a mistake. Exercise would lower Carrie's risk of illness, including heart disease, but wouldn't eliminate it. She still needed to pay attention to other disease risk factors, like dietary fat and smoking. Realizing that her entire family was increasing their risk of diseases such as high blood pressure, heart disease, and diabetes, Carrie convinced her sisters to join her in planning some food choices that were heart-healthier. Now, they still enjoy occasional burgers and chips, but have replaced the regular sodas with diet sodas, water, lemonade, and juice, and take turns bringing alternative offerings like grilled chicken, turkey burgers, and fresh fruit.

A Word on Counting Calories

I personally am not a fan of counting calories, but quite a few women feel that is the best way to for them to avoid overeating. For those who want to count calories, the current food labels provide plenty of information to keep those calculators humming. Just remember that gram for gram, carbohydrates and proteins provide the same number of calories, whereas fat packs more than twice as many.

One gram of this:	Has this number of calories:
Carbohydrate	4
Protein	4
Fat	9
Alcohol	7

THE FAT-FREE MYTH

Meg jogged several days each week and monitored her food intake very strictly. She complained that although her diet was almost "100 percent fat-free," she couldn't lose those last ten pounds.

Although Meg's situation was very different from Carrie's, she also needed to learn about moderation. She was exercising several days a week and paying close attention to her dietary fat intake. She had read a great deal about the importance of eating a low-fat diet, but like many women, she mistakenly believed that if low fat was good, no fat was even better. So Meg had tried to eliminate all fats from her diet. This left her diet too restricted in scope, so she was missing out on a lot of nutrients needed for optimal health. And not getting enough fat or variety led Meg to overindulge in fat-free snacks. What Meg failed to realize is the difference between *fat*-free and *calorie*-free: many of the snacks she ate were high in sugar and empty of nutrients. Without realizing it, Meg was eating approximately 500 calories a day in fat-free snack foods, which sabotaged her weight-loss efforts and reduced some of the health benefits she was getting from exercise.

Fat. Such a small word to provoke a huge amount of negative thoughts and feelings. Meg, like many women, equated dietary fat with body fat. She believed that avoiding the former would protect her from the latter. But excess body fat is formed when extra calories from *any source* are added to the body's storage tanks. And both dietary fat and body fat are not always the villains they are made out to be.

BODY COMPOSITION: MAKING A CASE AGAINST THE SCALE

Listening to some women talk about their bodies, I realize that many don't seem to understand that their bodies are composed of many tissues, of which fat is just one type. Even in very heavy women, *fat is not the predominant tissue* from which the human body is constructed. Ask anyone who has ever taken a junior-high-school science class, and they can tell you that *water* accounts for roughly two-thirds of body weight. The bones that make up the skeleton, and the tissues of the heart, brain, liver, kidneys, skin, and other organs also make a significant contribution to a woman's total weight. But it seems that even though fat is not the predominant *tissue,* it is the predominant *issue.* Too many women think that there is no such thing as good fat, but they're wrong.

Fat is an absolutely essential part of our bodies. It helps to form the brain, spinal cord, and nerves. It cushions the kidneys and other internal organs, and helps protect us from the cold. It can convert weak hormones into a usable form of estrogen. And it serves as a reservoir of energy that we can call on whenever we need it. Most women have no idea how convenient this really is. Your body routinely monitors available levels of energy, and will start taking fat out of storage as soon as it needs it, whether to sustain you during an exercise session, a shopping trip, or a life-threatening illness.

The key is to have the right amount of body fat—not too much, not too little. Women need about three times the amount of body fat as men, primarily for hormonal and reproductive purposes. Expressed as a percentage of total body weight, a woman's body needs enough fat to account for a bare minimum of 12 to 13 percent of her weight, or essential body functions will suffer. Similarly, if the percentage of body fat is more than twice as high as it needs to be, the risk of diseases associated with being overweight (and overfat) increases.

So either too much or too little fat impairs your body's ability to function properly and increases your susceptibility to disease. But too many women fixate on the number on the bathroom scale, because they mistakenly think of it as a way to measure their body fat. The irony is that the bathroom scale is a poor measurement of *anything,* including body fat. Even worse, some women see the scale as a tool for measuring self-worth, self-esteem, and health. Some of the young women I see weigh themselves several times each day, and they can't seem to grasp the fact that any change registered on the scale is nothing more than a reflection of water weight gained or lost throughout the day!

Think thin means healthy?

Think again. Some young women suffering from eating disorders may appear thin and healthy, but their cholesterol profiles tell a different story. These young women often have very high levels of cholesterol, indicating the body's distress at the lack of available energy sources. They also frequently complain of having *hypoglycemia,* or low blood sugar, when in reality they are in a state similar to early diabetes: their bodies have trouble processing carbohydrates because they eat them so erratically.

Contrary to our tendency to equate "thin" and "healthy," these women suffering from eating disorders are among the least healthy patients I see!

If you want to follow a number, it makes more sense to have your *body composition* determined. Body composition is a measurement of the relative percentages of lean tissue and fat for any given individual. Although body composition is considered to be a component of total fitness, I believe its measurement should be an issue of individual choice. For women who are motivated to exercise and eat healthfully if they have a number to follow, then periodic measurement of body composition is a good technique to follow. But for women who have a tendency to become enslaved by numbers, like their dress size or what appears on the bathroom scale, it can unwittingly become just another number to obsess over.

So decide for yourself. If you find that having a number to work toward helps you stick to your exercise program, by all means, have your body composition measured. One of my patients, Mona, was frustrated that although she exercised and "ate right," she always weighed ten pounds more than her younger sister. But when they joined a gym together and had their body fat measurements taken, Mona was amazed to find that her body fat was in the healthy range, but her sister's was too high to be considered healthy. For Mona, learning that her body's amount of fat was neither too high nor too low made her realize how much time she had wasted fretting over the number on the scale.

Why does it seem easy to lose weight quickly in the first week of a diet, but is so hard after that?
During the first few days of a diet, we tend to lose "water weight," which causes the number on the scale to drop fairly quickly. Fat loss occurs more slowly, over weeks to months, which takes time to show up on the scale. I recommend women focus on exercise and a healthy diet, and ignore the scale—the weight *will* come off, but gradually. If you insist on weighing yourself, don't weigh more frequently than once every one or two weeks, and follow the *trend* of the numbers downward rather than focusing on a specific number.

There are several methods for determining body composition, none of which are 100 percent accurate. Test results can vary widely and are influenced by many different factors, including the experience of the tester, dehydration, premenstrual bloating, and individual fat patterns. One of the simplest techniques for determining body composition utilizes skinfold calipers, which are most reliable in the hands of an experienced tester. A health care professional such as an exercise physiologist or nutritionist will probably give you the most accurate reading, but this test can be reliable when done by an experienced fitness professional as well. Keep in mind, though, that a hastily obtained measurement, poorly calibrated calipers, or an inexperienced tester can easily leave you with an inaccurate body fat measurement.

If you are interested in having your body fat measured, this is a relatively inexpensive and convenient method. It should not be measured more frequently than once every two or three months, but if you've started an exercise program with the goal of weight loss, it allows you to see concrete evidence that your body fat is decreasing. This is especially important if you are weight training, because adding muscle can make the number on the scale go up, not down.

Several of my patients have bought the recently introduced home scales that provide measurements of body weight and body fat. These work through bioelectrical impedance, a type of technology that is influenced greatly by an individual's state of hydration. The reliability of this technique is also influenced by a variety of other factors, like body position when the measurement is taken. For these reasons, I don't recommend these scales; I have not found their body fat determinations to be dependable. If you choose to use such a home device for body fat determination, be aware that any factors that influence the amount of water in your body, including a hard workout, alcohol, premenstrual bloating, and a recently eaten meal, can all affect the reading you get by as much as 30 percent!

There are several other methods, including underwater weighing and dual energy X-ray absorptiometry (DEXA; the same method widely used to determine bone density), which are used by researchers and are thought to be the most accurate. Since these techniques use very expensive pieces of equipment, they are most often used as research tools at universities and are not available to the general public. If you are interested in these techniques, check with a hospital, university, or medical school near you.

Body Composition Comparisons

Appearance	*Women (% body fat)*	*Men (% body fat)*
Very thin/skinny or a muscular elite athlete	Less than 17%	Less than 10%
Lean, but not skinny	17 to 21%	10 to 15%
Average, healthy appearing	21 to 26%	15 to 18%
Plump	26 to 33%	18 to 25%
Obese	33% or more	25% or more

While I believe that body composition measurements are the most helpful guide for weight loss, there are several other techniques in use by corporations, fitness professionals, and insurance companies that can be helpful. Each has benefits and limitations. These include:

> Body mass index, or BMI. This number is arrived at through the following mathematical equation:
>
> BMI = body weight in kilograms (kg) divided by the square of the height in meters (m). (One kilogram is equal to 2.2 pounds, and one meter is 39.6 inches.) For instance, the BMI for a 5'5" woman weighing 165 pounds is 28.
>
> BMI = 75 kg (165 pounds divided by 2.2) divided by 2.7 m (5'5" = 65 inches; 65 inches divided by 39.6 = 1.64 m; 1.64 m squared = 2.7).

BMI is thought to correlate with body composition more closely than weight alone does, but its critics argue that it does not take muscle mass into consideration. In general, a BMI of 25 or less is most desirable. A BMI greater than 30 is associated with obesity and increased risk of medical problems.

- *Waist-Hip ratio.* You have probably heard the "fruit theory" of weight-associated diseases: Those who carry excess fat around the middle (the "apples") have greater risk of weight-related medical problems than those who carry excess weight on the hips and thighs (the "pears"). If your waist measurement is more than 80 to 85 percent of your hip measurement (95 percent for men), you are considered an "apple." Although your risk of diabetes and heart disease is higher, you will find it easier to lose this excess fat than if it were deposited around the hips, thighs, and buttocks of the "pear."

- *Height and weight tables.* Although I think these are the least useful, many insurance companies continue to rely on height and weight for determining health risk. I use these on occasion to estimate a healthy weight *range* for patients. A reasonable guideline for women is 100 pounds for the first five feet of height, and 5 pounds per inch thereafter, plus or minus 10 percent. This gives me a general range to work with, which I find particularly helpful when dealing with an *underweight* patient. I add 10 percent if the patient is either big-boned or muscular, and subtract 10 percent of she is small-boned. For example, when I was treating a thin-appearing young woman who weighed 103 pounds at 5'4", I was able to use this guideline to *estimate* a healthy weight range of 110 to 130 pounds. Because she had an average bone structure, neither large nor small, we narrowed this range to 115 to 125, and chose an initial weight-gain goal of 10 to 15 pounds to maximize her sports performance and optimize her health. I emphasize *estimate,* because it is so important to remember that a tremendous number of variables affect the healthy weight range for each individual.

CHAPTER 9

HOW TO EAT LIKE AN ATHLETE

HIGH PROTEIN, low fat, single food, no sugar, no snacks, fat-burning, blood type, body type, and no carbs: just some of the most recent popular diet plans my patients have tried. Whether they are athletes or not, I encourage them to ignore the hype and follow the same sound nutrition principles with which sports nutritionists have been winning for years. Whether you are eating to prepare your body for a softball game, a marathon, or a morning at the beach with your kids, following a few basic dietary principles will help you successfully fuel your muscles for maximum energy. If you are an active woman, paying attention to getting enough of the "right" types of fuel will help you successfully reach the goals of your exercise program. Even more important, learning to eat like an athlete can ultimately improve your overall health.

FOOD AS FUEL

Judging from the tremendous number of eating plans, diets, and supplements endorsed by athletes and other celebrities, it's easy to develop the impression that eating right is a confusing, sophisticated equation. The truth is, however, that eating to fuel your life in general, and your exercise performance in particular, couldn't be easier. You don't need a Ph.D. in nutrition—just a knowledge of the basics and a dose of common sense.

Fuel, or food as we more commonly call it, falls into one of three basic categories: carbohydrate, protein, or fat. You can think of these three basic categories of fuel for the human body in the same way you might think of gasoline, electricity, or oil: each has its own benefits and limitations as a power source. Many people refer to specific foods as "bad" or "good," but in reality all food is just fuel. Some is premium quality, some has lots of additives; some is cheap, some is expensive; some is abundant, some is scarce. None of these factors affect the fact that food is just fuel.

What these factors do affect, however, is how efficiently your body is able to use and store the energy provided by the foods you eat. This is most obvious when you exercise, because exercise requires the presence of fairly large quantities of fuel. In general, carbohydrates provide the best source of calories for exercise, because carbohydrates are the easiest source of fuel for the muscles to use. That's why most nutritionists recommend that 50 to 60 percent of your dietary intake comes from carbohydrates. Once ingested, carbohydrates are broken down into glucose; the glucose is either burned for fuel immediately or stored as glycogen in the muscles and liver, where it is readily accessible. Once your muscle and liver glycogen stores are stuffed, excess carbohydrates will eventually be stored as body fat.

Fat can also be used as fuel, but only after a complicated digestion process during which the body repackages it in a more easily used form. Unfortunately, while less than efficient at using dietary fat for fuel, the body is very efficient at storing dietary fat as energy reserves. Once stored as body fat, this fuel isn't as easily accessed by the exercising muscles, but the longer you exercise, the more time your muscles have to get this source of energy out of storage so it can be used. That's why women who want to lose weight need to have exercise sessions longer than those whose exercise goals are purely health related.

It's important to know that although the muscles can use fat as an energy source, they need some glucose around to function well. In addition, the brain won't settle for fat, but rather demands glucose for energy. For these reasons, dieters who try to avoid eating glucose-supplying carbohydrates with the hope of burning fat stores instead will fail. Such a plan will ultimately leave you feeling exhausted, clumsy, and without the mental power to stay committed to your exercise plan.

The third type of fuel, protein, can be used to provide energy for exercise, but your body won't be too happy about it. It prefers to save protein for other uses, such as building and repairing muscle tissue and constructing new cells and hormones. A common misconception is that women who participate in weight training have a greater need for dietary protein. Generally, that's not true. Whether your favorite activity is lifting weights, running, playing soccer, or practicing yoga, your muscles prefer carbohydrates for energy. Only a small amount of protein is actually needed to provide enough raw material for the building and repairing process that takes place in muscles undergoing weight training.

It doesn't take much to fulfill your daily need for protein. No matter how much protein you choose to eat, there is a limit to how much your body is able to use. And just like with fat and excess carbohydrates, your body stores excess protein as fat—not as muscle, as some advocates of high protein diets would have you believe. For most women, four to six ounces of protein daily meets their bodies' requirements. (For reference, a piece of fish or meat the size of a deck of cards is three to four ounces.)

Of course, if you limit the total amount of calories you consume, your diet may be deficient in all three fuel sources. This is a situation I encounter frequently when dealing with an athlete with recurrent or chronic injuries. Adequate nutrients, including sufficient total calories, protein, and vitamins C and E have been implicated as critical, often overlooked, elements of the injury healing process. So food not only fuels your exercise program, it helps fuel your ability to get healthy and stay that way!

Type of Fuel	What It's Used For	Where to Get It
Carbohydrate	Brain function Muscle energy	Vegetables, fruits, pasta, rice, breads, cereal
Fat	Sustained or low-level activity	Vegetable oils (including olive oil); animal fats (such as meat and butter)
Protein	Building and repairing the body's tissues, including muscles, blood cells, and hormones	Fish, poultry and other meats, eggs, beans, dairy products, nuts

Does it matter how soon I eat after a workout?
That depends. After exercise, your muscles refuel with glycogen, a storage form of carbohydrate. Carbohydrate is stored more rapidly if eaten within two hours after a workout. If you're training twice a day, or if you are one of an increasing number of women taking an active vacation that involves several hours of activity a day, it's a good idea to eat a carbohydrate-rich meal or snack within two hours of completing your activity. But for the rest of us who are exercising once a day or less, the timing of your next meal or snack isn't crucial.

A NEW LOOK AT THE FOOD PYRAMID

Most of us have seen the government's recommended food pyramid (below), which appears on packages of many different types of food, including cereal and crackers.

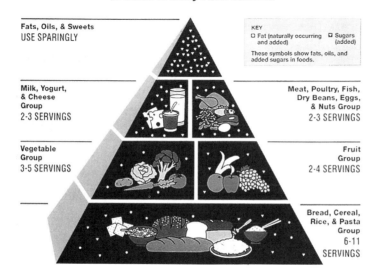

Food Guide Pyramid
A Guide to Daily Food Choices

Fats, Oils, & Sweets
USE SPARINGLY

KEY
□ Fat (naturally occurring and added)   □ Sugars (added)
These symbols show fats, oils, and added sugars in foods.

Milk, Yogurt, & Cheese Group
2-3 SERVINGS

Meat, Poultry, Fish, Dry Beans, Eggs, & Nuts Group
2-3 SERVINGS

Vegetable Group
3-5 SERVINGS

Fruit Group
2-4 SERVINGS

Bread, Cereal, Rice, & Pasta Group
6-11 SERVINGS

Sports nutritionists typically recommend that 60 percent of your dietary intake should come in the form of carbohydrate, about 25 percent from fat, and 15 percent from protein. Now, here's where a lot of my patients have gone wrong: They realize that carbohydrates are found in starches, including breads, pasta, and grains. But they don't realize that carbohydrates are also found in the sugars and starches of fruits and vegetables. Relying on bread, bagels, and pasta as the only sources of carbohydrate, and ignoring fruits and vegetables, has caused many well-intentioned women to end up eating *more* calories than their bodies need. This is largely because foods like bagels and pasta are more likely to be eaten along with fats, like butter and cream. But it's also due to confusion over what constitutes a portion.

The pyramid's base layer recommends 6 to 11 servings of carbohydrate in the form of grains, rice, cereal, breads, and pasta. But what we may think of as 1 serving is often much more. Our food culture is so "supersized" that we don't even realize how much we're actually eating every day. For instance, a typical deli bagel is not 1 or 2 servings of carbohydrate; it's actually 4 servings! So a bagel for breakfast and a sandwich at lunchtime could satisfy the pyramid's recommended grain intake for the entire day. In addition, minimizing fruits and vegetables as important sources of carbohydrate means missing out in some critically important nutrients. Learning to eat well for health, weight control, and athletic performance means taking a careful look not only at *what* is on your plate, but *how much* is there.

That being said, I don't think most people need to worry about measuring everything they eat. You'll be in the ballpark if you do the following:

- Familiarize yourself with the food pyramid
- Remember that fruits and vegetables are important carbohydrates
- Read labels for nutritional content, not just calorie counting
- Learn to recognize appropriate serving sizes
- Pay attention to what and how much you're actually eating

FEMALE ATHLETES AND THE VEGETARIAN DIET

Often, a female athlete will tell me that she's a vegetarian, when what she really means is she doesn't eat meat. There's no doubt that a diet exclusive of meat can be a healthy one, as long as you get adequate protein from nonmeat sources—and as long as calling yourself "vegetarian" isn't just a cover for disordered eating (see the section on The Female Athlete Triad in chapter 10).

Protein supplies *amino acids,* which are the actual building blocks your body needs to repair and build various tissues. Your body can make some of these amino acids, but eight of them (the so-called *essential* amino acids) must come from food. All of these essential amino acids are present in some protein sources, like dairy and soy products, meat, fish, and chicken. Other protein sources, like beans, rice, and nuts, have low levels of some of these critical building blocks. If you are vegetarian, it's important that you eat a large enough variety of foods so that you get adequate amounts of all the essential amino acids. However, contrary to conventional wisdom, you don't have to eat special combinations of foods to get all the essential amino acids in one meal, you just need to be sure your daily diet includes them all.

WATER, WATER, EVERYWHERE

While water is not a type of fuel, it is a critically important nutrient. You can live much longer without food than without water. Many women are chronically dehydrated and don't realize it, because the symptoms of dehydration are so subtle. They complain of being "tired all the time" or "not having any energy." And it's no wonder when you stop to think about all the body's functions that require water. Water is the main component of blood, so it's responsible for pushing oxygen and nutrients on to be delivered to working tissues; it carries waste products away from cells and flushes them through the kidneys. Many of the chemical reactions that keep your metabolism humming need a constant supply of water.

Most women are familiar with the recommendation of drinking eight glasses of water a day, but many don't realize this applies to the average day in the life of a sedentary woman. Some recent research has suggested that eight glasses isn't enough, even for the most sedentary of women. Those researchers suggested multiplying your weight by .04, then doubling the result to find your own water needs. For instance, for a women weighing 150 pounds, the following equation would apply:

$$150 \times .04 = 6$$
$$6 \times 2 = 12 \text{ glasses of water}$$

While this has not replaced conventional wisdom, I do think it makes sense that a larger woman needs a larger volume of water. Try gradually increasing your water intake and see how you feel. And remember, when you increase your activity through exercise, your need for water increases as well. Occasionally, an athlete or patient tells me she doesn't like water, in which case I recommend she increase her intake of water through a variety of fluids, including juice, seltzer, and herbal teas, or water-filled foods, like lettuce, cucumbers, tomatoes, and fruits such as watermelon or grapefruit.

You can lose a great deal of water through exercise before you become thirsty, which will affect your performance. How can you prevent this from happening? There are formulas you can follow, such as the recommendation to drink a cup of water for every fifteen to twenty minutes of exercise. Or you can weigh yourself before and after exercise and drink two to three cups of water for every pound of water loss during exercise. The simplest method is to monitor the color and volume of your urine: when it's plentiful, clear, and pale yellow, you're well hydrated. When it's scanty and dark yellow to golden, you are dehydrated and need to drink water until your urine becomes pale again. Be aware, however, that if you are taking vitamins, supplements, or certain medications that affect the color of your urine, this may not be a reliable way for you to monitor your state of hydration.

What to Drink?

Conventional wisdom is that if you are exercising for less than an hour, water is all you need for fluid intake, but if you are exercising for more than an hour, you need fluids like sports drinks, which provide a quick source of energy. You can buy prepared commercial sports drinks, or make your own by diluting one ounce of juice with four or five ounces of water.

During exercise, try to drink cold water, as it is absorbed more quickly. It also helps to cool you off, because muscles work so hard during exercise that they cause the entire body to heat up. Even if you're exercising in very cold weather, you still need fluids, although you may want to consider getting them from a warmer source, like herbal tea, hot chocolate, or broth. And remember, drinks containing caffeine and alcohol don't work for fluid replacement. They increase fluid loss through the kidneys, making it more likely that you will become dehydrated.

TAKING IT TO THE NEXT LEVEL: THE GLYCEMIC INDEX

Many athletes make food choices based on the *glycemic index.* The glycemic index of any specific food is determined by how quickly that particular food is digested, which is affected by many variables, including the way it's prepared and how much fiber it contains. Foods that are digested quickly are said to have a high glycemic index, whereas those that are broken down more slowly have a low glycemic index. In general, the more rapidly a food is digested, the more quickly it contributes glucose (blood sugar) into the circulation. Initially, doctors and nutritionists thought they could use this concept to try to help people with diabetes control their blood sugars. It became somewhat impractical when it was realized that during a meal, when several different foods are eaten at the same time, the glycemic index of any one food is unimportant.

But athletes quickly realized that this concept could help them choose the right snacks to fuel their activity. Eating a low glycemic index food *before* exercise ensures a slow release of glucose into the bloodstream, which many athletes have found helps sustain their energy during exercise. If an athlete needs a quick source of energy *during* exercise, a high glycemic index food is a better choice, because it enters the bloodstream rapidly, supplying glucose for quick energy. And you don't have to be an elite athlete to benefit from this approach. Making food choices based on their glycemic index can help women sustain a high level of energy throughout the day.

I have found that understanding the concept of glycemic index is especially helpful for women who exercise late in the day. Many times, late-day exercisers are tired, and they choose foods like candy bars, graham crackers, or jelly beans (all high glycemic) to help power them through their exercise session. Often they complain they're ravenous afterward. This can be a problem, especially if postexercise hunger frequently draws you to the cookie jar for a quick fix. But lower glycemic index foods, like a handful of dried apricots or low-fat fruit yogurt, supply energy over a longer period of time, and can prevent that postexercise cookie-jar raid.

How do you find the right snack for you? Experiment! There is no right choice for everyone. What and when you choose to snack is just as much an individual choice as designing your exercise program. For instance, I personally have found low-fat chocolate milk or a banana to be my favorite pre-workout foods, but I know athletes who do better with a glass of orange juice, a sweet potato, or a cup of popcorn. Give foods from the following chart a try, and see what works for you.

High Glycemic Index Foods	Medium Glycemic Index Foods	Low Glycemic Index Foods
Gatorade	Orange juice	Milk
Candy bar	Ripe banana	Underripe banana
Baked potato	Sweet potato	Pear
Rice cakes	Rice	PowerBar
Jelly beans	Popcorn	Low-fat fruit yogurt
Bagel	Bran muffin	Apple
Raisins	Orange	Grapefruit
Oatmeal	Bran cereal	Barley

Snacking on the Go

Being prepared for snack attacks will help you stick to a smart, healthy eating plan. Although some women worry that snacks are unnecessary sources of calories, they have a place in a well-balanced diet. It's much smarter to take the edge off hunger with a quick snack than to let your blood sugar plummet as your hunger builds, which will leave you feeling weak, irritable, and more likely to reach for a quick fix from a high-sugar, high-fat food.

Carry an emergency supply of a nonperishable snack in your purse, briefcase, or gym bag, and don't wait until you are ravenous to eat it. Try keeping a Baggie filled with a favorite cereal, animal crackers, pretzels, or nuts mixed with raisins or other dried fruit on hand, so you'll have a healthy alternative to the ubiquitous high-fat, high-sugar, low-nutrient offerings of the vending machine. Be creative: Buy several different varieties of nuts and dried fruit, and try different combinations. Try a handful of soy nuts, chopped walnuts, dried cranberries, and mango; or peanuts, slivered almonds, dried papaya, and apricots. The possibilities are endless!

And if you're caught unprepared and find yourself faced with fast-food options for a quick meal, remember to seek out the carbohydrates. One of the smartest fast-food choices you can make is a slice of pizza, especially if it's topped with extra veggies and low-fat cheese. But ignore the subtle appeal of thin crust and opt for the thick crust, because thin crust gets more calories from fat, whereas thick crust provides more carbohydrates. Other good choices for high-carbohydrate, low-fat grab-and-go meals or snacks include these:

- turkey or roast beef submarine sandwich, no mayonnaise
- waffles with fruit

CARBO-LOADING

Athletes training for a marathon, triathlon, or other endurance sporting event have long known about carbo-loading, a carbohydrate-rich eating plan that stuffs the muscles full of energy-providing glycogen in anticipation of the big event. But many don't realize that proper carbo-loading doesn't mean just eating pasta and bread for a day or two before the event. To effectively load the muscles with glycogen, you must start at least three weeks before your race, and eat enough carbohydrates to account for 60 to 70 percent of your daily nutrient intake. It's also important to get enough protein, so you'll need to skimp on fats in favor of both carbs and protein. Simple switches like jam instead of butter on toast, or low-fat yogurt instead of ice cream will help you meet this goal.

Be warned, however, that the main downside to carbo-loading is gastrointestinal distress. More carbs and less fats means more volume of food, which can lead to stomach upset. If this happens to you, try spacing your intake throughout the day in four or five meals. Trying to carbo-load with lots of fruit can cause abdominal cramps and diarrhea. Last but not least, be sure your water intake is adequate, or carbo-loading might lead to constipation.

- bean burrito with salsa
- chili with beans and rice
- baked potato with broccoli and low-fat cheese

VITAMINS AND MINERALS: FOOD FIRST!

Melody was a collegiate gymnast who came to see me because she was always tired. Her workouts were suffering, and she was worried about losing her spot on the team. She was hoping I could recommend a vitamin or supplement to give her an energy boost.

Melody reported that she had a tendency to develop bulky thighs, so since high school she had followed the advice of her coach to avoid bread, potatoes, and pasta. As a result, her diet lacked enough energy-rich carbohydrates. No wonder she was tired! When I explained this to Melody, she looked at me and sighed. "But I don't want to gain weight," she said. "Can't you just give me a vitamin or something?"

Melody's question is a common one. But despite the advertisements that have helped make supplements a multi-million-dollar industry, vitamins and minerals are *not* a source of energy. They are a vitally important presence in the human body, without which many chemical reactions cannot occur. They help in building and repairing the body's infrastructure and constantly assist in numerous important functions. Without them, your body suffers. But only the three substances the body uses as fuel—carbohydrate, fat, and protein—can provide energy.

There is controversy over whether or not vitamins and minerals in pill form are as well absorbed as those in foods. Even if there is no significant difference in vitamin absorption, food has other benefits that make it superior to pills for providing the nutrients women need for optimal health. For instance, many women shun calcium in milk in favor of taking it in the form of a supplement. But by ignoring milk, they are missing a valuable source of protein, potassium, and phosphorus. Milk is also an excellent source of *riboflavin* (a B vitamin), which is a critical catalyst for the chemical reactions that convert food into usable energy. And since riboflavin is one of the vitamins active women need more of than do sedentary women, milk is a particularly wise choice for active women to include in their diets.

A final note: There is so much we just don't know about the health-enhancing benefits of most foods. Although no new vitamins have been recently discovered, new health benefits of specific foods are constantly being reported. Take, for example, the recognition that *lycopene,* a recently discovered phytochemical found in tomatoes, is a potent soldier in the battle against cancer. If you have been relying

SHOULD I TAKE A VITAMIN/MINERAL SUPPLEMENT?

The answer: It depends. If your diet typically has plenty of variety and an adequate number of calories, you probably get enough vitamins and minerals from your food. Many women, even if they feel their diet is adequate, like to take a multivitamin as "extra insurance" to be sure they are meeting all their vitamin and mineral requirements. That seems to be a safe practice, but remember that more isn't always better. Your body stores vitamins, so even if your diet is not as nutritious on some days as others, you'll have vitamin reserves to dip into. If you take more vitamins than your body wants, your kidneys will excrete most excess amounts. But some vitamins, particularly A, D, E, and K, will continue stockpiling in your body's fat cells, with dangerous consequences. Similarly, excess minerals like iron can cause organ damage and may even increase your risk of a heart attack.

If you suspect there are deficiencies in your diet, ask a nutritionist to evaluate your typical intake and make recommendations. Don't just start experimenting with supplements on your own, or you could end up in much worse shape than you started in.

on supplements, you've been missing out because no supplements contain this recently discovered, naturally occurring compound found in plants. So avoid the temptation to swallow a pill, and remember, when it comes to maximizing your health, think "food first!"

CREATINE, CAFFEINE, AND OTHER SUPPLEMENTS

Searching for the perfect performance-enhancing aid has long been a part of elite-level competitive athletics. But more and more recreational athletes are experimenting with steroids and nutritional supplements, searching for the same edge. Women are not immune to this phenomenon. One study showed that while anabolic steroid use is declining among high-school boys, it's increasing among teenage girls! Many women come into my office asking questions about the supplements touted to enhance athletic performance that are front and center in many local pharmacies. But do they work?

The answer: Yes, no, it depends, and we don't know. Because herbs and supplements are not regulated by the FDA, there is little controlled research about the safety and efficacy of most of the pills and powders popular with athletes. Many of the claims made about these substances are from research done by the companies that make them, not exactly an unbiased source of information. When you are trying to evaluate a claim made about a particular substance, look for research done on real athletes, not rats or other lab animals; don't get wowed by testimonials and pictures of hard bodies in skimpy bathing suits; and always check with your doctor before taking anything new. Many supplements are probably harmless, but some have ingredients that can be life-threatening. Case in point: Those containing ephedra, or ephedrine, an adrenaline-like compound sold as an energy booster and weight-loss aid. Also seen as *ma huang,* this ingredient can cause heart palpitations, exacerbate high blood pressure, and has been linked to several deaths.

I have been surprised by the number of women who are interested in trying creatine, one of the most popular supplements in recent years. A naturally occurring compound found in meat and fish, creatine is used by muscles for quick bursts of energy. It has been taken primarily by male athletes in sports like football, in which there are brief, intense bursts of activity. The only group of my female patients who have liked taking this supplement are the competitive body-builders. The other female athletes in my practice have all been turned off by the weight gain that accompanies the use of this supplement. (It's thought that this is water-weight gain, but the jury is still out.) Creatine is thought to be safe, but no long-term studies have been completed yet.

Finally, many of my patients are so used to their morning cups of java that they are amazed to learn that caffeine is a stimulant popular with athletes, especially recreational ones. Many competitive athletes avoid caffeine, especially precompetition, because it makes them feel jittery. However, some studies of cyclists have shown that caffeine prolongs the length of time they can exercise before their muscles fatigue. And a number of recreational athletes, especially women, tell me they can't exercise without it. Why is this? Probably because caffeine has a stimulant effect on the brain, so they feel less fatigued and are more easily able to complete their exercise sessions. *But more is not necessarily better!* In addition to causing jitters, caffeine's stimulant effect can make your pulse race and cause stomach upset. Worse, it's a diuretic and can contribute to dehydration. High levels of caffeine (the amount you'd get in four or five large cups of coffee or sixteen cola drinks) in the blood of an Olympic athlete will lead to disqualification, even though there's no proof that large amounts of caffeine boost performance. If you feel that you need a mild stimulant to get you going in your exercise session, consider sniffing peppermint: a couple of interesting studies have concluded that simply smelling peppermint can make you feel more energetic and ready to exercise.

SPECIAL NUTRITIONAL REQUIREMENTS FOR FEMALE ATHLETES

Calcium

Calcium is a particularly important mineral in the diet of active women. Although most people think of calcium as having a vital role in building healthy bones, it is in high demand for multiple additional functions, including muscle contraction, blood pressure regulation, and hormone secretion. It has also been found to have a role in reducing symptoms of PMS. As we learn more and more about the varied roles of calcium, we realize it is one of the most important minerals in the human body.

Because there has been a great deal of attention paid to the fact that exercise is important for the prevention of osteoporosis, many young women mistakenly believe that they do not need to worry about calcium intake as long as they exercise. Not so! No amount of exercise will compensate for the lack of calcium and other nutrients needed to build strong bones. In fact, young women who exercise intensely enough to lose their menstrual cycles are at greater risk for osteoporosis to develop prematurely. (For more about premature osteoporosis, see the section on the female athlete triad in chapter 10).

Because women have thinner and lighter bones than men, their calcium reservoir is smaller, so it's critical that dietary intake of calcium be maximized. The current RDI (Recommended Daily Intake) of calcium for women over eighteen years of age is 1,000 to 1,500 mgs. While dairy products are the best known sources of calcium, dark-green vegetables, soy products, and canned fish like sardines and salmon (you must eat the bones for these to count!) also provide some calcium. Many young women are surprised to learn that cream cheese is a poor source of calcium, with only 23 milligrams in 1 ounce (2 tablespoons).

To get enough dietary calcium usually means 3 to 4 servings of the following each day:

1 cup of milk, yogurt, pudding, or calcium-fortified orange juice
1.5 ounces of cheese
2 cups of cottage cheese
1.5 cups of cooked spinach
1.5 to 2 cups of broccoli or dark-green leafy vegetables
1.5 cups of milk-based frozen yogurt

Iron

Iron is the most abundant metal in the body. Although small amounts are stored in the bone marrow, it's found primarily in circulating red blood cells, where it helps form hemoglobin, the molecule responsible for the transport and delivery of oxygen. Small amounts of iron are lost daily through sweat, and through shedding of old cells from the skin and the lining of the gastrointestinal tract. It is blood loss, however, through monthly menstruation that is the biggest cause of iron depletion, resulting in *iron-deficiency anemia.* This means that the body's ability to deliver oxygen to its cells is diminished, leading to the most common symptom of anemia, fatigue.

Doctors and nutritionists have long known that women who are vegetarians frequently don't get enough iron in their diets, and that they are particularly at risk for developing this common ailment. But it is less well recognized that iron-deficiency anemia is also common in active women, whether or not they eat meat. It is unclear why, although many experts believe it is simply because too many women don't eat *enough of anything.* It is estimated that the average woman needs to eat between 2,000 and 3,000 calories each day to get the recommended amount of dietary iron, but many women are watching their weight, and don't get more than half the recommended number of calories. Other factors that may contribute to anemia in active women include the use of anti-inflammatory medications, like ibuprofen and naproxen, which have been linked to slow, microscopic "leaks" of blood from the intestinal lining. While this blood loss is not enough to be life-threatening, it can lead to gradually diminished iron stores and iron-deficiency anemia.

Although only a small amount of iron is usually required daily in the diet, once a woman has developed iron-deficiency anemia, she needs significantly more daily iron than usual, so she can replenish her iron stores. Fortunately, simply taking an iron supplement for a few months will do the trick. Iron supplements are available without a doctor's prescription, but a word of caution: Iron supplements should be taken only under a doctor's supervision, after a blood test has confirmed the correct diagnosis. Too much iron can cause damage to the liver and has even recently become suspected of contributing to heart disease. If you think you need to take an iron supplement, check with your doctor first!

To maximize the iron in your diet:

- Eat a couple of ounces of lean beef or pork, or the dark meat of chicken or turkey. In addition to being terrific sources of iron, these meats provide protein and zinc. (As your mother knew, liver is a great source of iron—but it's also full of cholesterol! Try these lean, heart-friendlier cuts of meat instead.)
- Other good sources of iron include iron-fortified cereals and breads (vegetable sources of iron, like broccoli, aren't very well absorbed).
- Eat iron-rich foods and vitamin C at the same time, because vitamin C helps you absorb dietary iron.
- Don't drink coffee and tea at the same time you're eating your iron-rich food, because they will decrease the amount of iron you absorb.
- Try cooking in cast-iron pots: some will leach into your food.

CHAPTER 10

EATING DISORDERS, DISORDERED EATING, AND THE FEMALE ATHLETE TRIAD

MOST OF US THINK athletes are models of good health—and good health habits. There's a common tendency to think that active women not only know more about nutrition, but that they can—and do—eat whatever they want without worrying about excess weight gain. But unfortunately, athletic women are no more immune to cultural pressures to be thin than are the rest of us. Ironically, even some of the most elite athletes—those we admire for their hard-earned skills and envy for their lean looks—feel the most pressure to appear slender. This constant focus on appearance leads many active and athletic women to develop unhealthy, even dangerous, attitudes toward food and their bodies. The result can be a full-blown eating disorder—or, much more commonly, an approach toward food called *disordered eating.*

EATING DISORDERS

Many people are at least somewhat familiar with the eating disorders known to the public as *anorexia* and *bulimia*. The formal medical names of these two disorders, *anorexia nervosa* and *bulimia nervosa*, hint at the fact that these have long been recognized as specific psychiatric illnesses, which can affect anyone—even an athlete.

Anorexia Nervosa

Anorexia nervosa is thought to affect less than 1 percent of the population, with young women in late adolescence or early adulthood most frequently affected. Young women affected by anorexia nervosa have an intense, unreasonable fear of gaining weight. They suffer from a distorted body image, as if they were looking at a reflection in a funhouse mirror. A person with anorexia nervosa weighs less than 85 percent of what is considered normal for her age and height. Menstruation, if it ever began, ceases. And despite intense treatment, anorexia nervosa not infrequently results in death.

Bulimia Nervosa

Bulimia nervosa is estimated to be slightly more common than anorexia nervosa, affecting 1 to 3 percent of the population. In contrast to the emaciated appearance of the woman with anorexia nervosa, a sufferer of bulimia nervosa usually looks to be of normal weight. The hallmark of bulimia nervosa is recurrent episodes of *binge eating*. A binge is not just mindlessly eating a few cookies too many while watching your favorite sitcom. Rather, binge eating is medically defined as consuming an abnormally large amount of food in a limited period of time, during which the binger feels she has no control over the binge. Patients with bulimia nervosa try to prevent binge-associated weight gain by quickly inducing vomiting or diarrhea, fasting or exercising excessively to compensate for binges. This behavior becomes a pattern, with episodes of bingeing and compensatory behavior occurring at least twice a week for three months or more. Compared to anorexia nervosa, bulimia nervosa is less likely to result in death, but it's associated with numerous medical problems, like disturbances in the body's electrolytes, such as sodium and potassium, and erosion of dental enamel caused by self-induced vomiting.

DISORDERED EATING

Whereas both anorexia nervosa and bulimia nervosa are clearly recognized psychiatric conditions, disordered eating behavior is less well understood—and less frequently recognized. Ironically, disordered-eating patterns can be so common that they are erroneously viewed as "normal." Take, for instance, a patient of mine named Christina, a dance major at a local college. A Broadway hopeful with wide blue eyes and a megawatt smile, she spends several hours a day dancing: ballet, jazz, modern. A few months ago, one of her mentors took her aside and told her that she'd never have a chance of making it as a performer unless she dropped ten to fifteen pounds. Determined to lose weight, she stopped eating many of her favorite foods, like pasta, bread, and potatoes. Her diet became limited to dry cereal, salads, and cans of tuna. She avoided social occasions that involved food and began using an herbal laxative. Christina didn't stand out among her classmates; in fact, many of them had similar diets. However, in her efforts to lose weight, Christina had developed disordered eating.

The term *disordered eating* refers to a wide spectrum of unhealthy eating patterns that are, unfortunately, all too common among American girls and women, both athletes and nonathletes. Often, disordered eating begins when a young woman simply starts to monitor everything that she eats. She progresses to restricting certain foods; in my experience, this is usually meat (especially red meat) or sweets. By eliminating one food after another from her acceptable choices, she ends up with a severely limited diet. Choosing from her limited options means she eats the same foods repetitively.

In my medical practice, I've come to recognize several patterns of repetitive eating. An example of what I see most commonly: breakfast is nothing, or possibly half a bagel (often with the inside scooped out) or a handful of dry cereal; lunch is a salad; dinner is pasta with red sauce (no meat). Snacks, if allowed, are usually pretzels, occasionally a piece of fruit, or frozen yogurt (which I hear variably described as a "treat," or a forbidden snack eaten "when I'm being bad"). While clearly not anorexia or bulimia, such disordered eating lacks the nutritional punch ensured by variety, has minimal protein and fat, and falls short of supplying many critical nutrients, including iron and calcium. It also is so prevalent that parents, coaches, and teachers frequently don't recognize it as abnormal.

I've seen disordered-eating patterns among all ages, from an eleven-year-old tennis player to a seventy-year-old runner. It sometimes shows up in surprising ways, like one sixty-eight-year-old skier who refused to eat in the hospital after knee surgery because she couldn't exercise to get rid of the calories. Similarly, I remember a thirty-four-year-old new mother who wanted to breast-feed, but whose caloric intake was much too low for her body to produce breast milk. And I have seen too many women like Deborah, a forty-year-old runner with iron-deficiency anemia whose one meal each day was carrots, rice cakes, and peanut butter.

But disordered eating is not just about limiting calories or restricting specific foods. It may also include fasting; using diet pills, laxatives, or diuretics; and periodic bingeing and purging. In other words, many of the behaviors are the same as those involved in anorexia and bulimia, but they aren't as severe. Some experts believe that unchecked disordered-eating behavior can lead to the development of a full-blown eating disorder. Disordered eating can also be the first step toward development of the *female athlete triad.*

THE FEMALE ATHLETE TRIAD

About a decade ago, several of my astute colleagues began describing a common pattern they were observing among female athletes. They noticed that many active young women were drastically altering their diets, developing disordered-eating behavior in the hopes of improving their athletic success by becoming thinner. As a result, they were developing problems with their menstrual periods, ranging from skipping several in a row to stopping menstruation altogether (medically known as *amenorrhea,* meaning "no menstruation"). The doctors knew that such menstrual abnormalities meant the athletes had inadequate levels of estrogen, and worried that the low estrogen levels might prevent the young women from developing normal, healthy bones. Their fears were confirmed when they began testing the bone density of these athletes and found that many of them were developing premature osteoporosis. In 1993, they coined the term *female athlete triad* to describe this alarming association between disordered eating, amenorrhea, and osteoporosis. The triad often goes undetected; frequently it is not suspected until the athlete suffers a stress fracture similar to the type seen in postmenopausal women with osteoporosis.

Suzanne, one of my patients, fits the typical profile of the female athlete triad. A twenty-seven-year-old runner, she became a vegetarian, ostensibly for ethical reasons but secretly because she believed cutting meat and dairy from her diet would allow her to become thinner—and faster. She began to monitor everything she ate, avoiding fat in addition to meat and dairy products. A typical day's food intake was a banana for breakfast; lettuce, tomato and carrot salad for lunch; and beans and rice or stir-fried vegetables for dinner. She was proud of her new "healthy diet" and resulting weight loss. She lost something else, too—her period—but instead of being worried, she was thrilled: no period, no cramps. She continued running, adding a second workout at the gym on days she "felt fat," or on the rare occasion when she indulged her craving for sweets. She was referred to me by her gynecologist after her fourth stress fracture. A bone density test confirmed that Suzanne had osteoporosis, with the bone density of the average sixty-eight-year-old woman.

Who's at Risk for the Triad?

No one knows how prevalent the female athlete triad really is, but my experiences taking care of active and athletic women have convinced me that it's extremely common.

Initially it was recognized in athletes who participated in sports with subjective judging (like figure skating and gymnastics), those who needed to make weight (like in judo or lightweight rowing), or athletes participating in sports in which thinness was perceived as advantageous (like distance running). Now, however, young women suffering with the female athlete triad have been recognized in virtually all sports, including swimming, basketball, hockey, and boxing.

Surveys have reported that up to 62 percent of athletic women have eating patterns typical of disordered eating. Women who are generally thought to be at greatest risk are those who've been chronic dieters, have low self-esteem, come from dysfunctional families, have a history of abuse, and have perfectionist personalities. Risk increases during life changes when women might feel more vulnerable, such as when going off to college, or after a traumatic event like an injury.

Personally, I think disordered eating has more to do with "female" than "athlete"; that is to say, I don't believe that disordered eating is necessarily any more common among athletes than it is among women in general. However, amenorrhea seems to be more common among athletes than nonathletes, especially among dancers and runners. No one knows why this is, but many experts believe that it is due to the fact that athletes with inadequate diets burn more calories than they consume. In this scenario, the body doesn't have enough calories around to fuel all its processes, so it uses the available calories for its most necessary functions, like the workings of the brain and heart. There's not enough left over to fuel the reproductive system, so the menstrual cycle stops. From an evolutionary viewpoint, this makes perfect sense; if the body isn't getting enough energy (i.e., food) to maintain all its processes, it needs to go into survival mode. Why fuel the re-productive system—and, consequently, take a chance on get-ting pregnant—when there's not enough fuel (food) around for one, much less two?

Fortunately, this type of amenorrhea is reversible. Once the fuel deficit is corrected and there are enough calories available, the menstrual cycle usually resumes. All's well that ends well, some athletes think. But it's not that simple. No one knows whether this history of amenorrhea associ-ated with the female athlete triad affects future fertility. And very worrisome is the persistence of the third component of the triad, *premature osteoporosis.*

Although it's often thought of as a postmenopausal woman's disease, osteoporosis can occur in women of any age. This can be because of bone loss—or inadequate bone formation. Our bones should be rapidly developing, growing denser and stronger, from the time we begin menstruating dur-ing our teen years until our mid-twenties. Unfortunately, if a young woman is not menstruating as expected during this time, her bones don't develop optimally, which puts her at risk for premature osteoporosis. If that's not a frightening enough thought, consider this: Some studies suggest that this process of premature osteoporosis may be irreversible, even if disor-dered eating is corrected and periods resume. If further stud-ies show this is true, we may well have a generation of young women with the osteoporotic bones of their grandmothers!

Treating and Preventing the Triad

I'll be honest here: Treating the triad is tough. I have the "it takes a village" mentality toward treating the triad. The most effective treatment comes from a dedicated team of professionals, including a physician, nutritionist, mental health professional, and exercise physiologist; it frequently requires involvement of the athlete's coach and support system (like parents, team athletic trainer, and friends).

Ultimately, our goal should be to prevent, rather than treat, the female athlete triad. Preventing the triad depends first and foremost upon education—of athletes, parents, and coaches. We need to dispel a couple of common misconceptions. First, while anorexia tends to be fairly dramatic and easy to recognize, disordered eating is not. Coaches and parents need to realize that just because an athlete doesn't look anorexic doesn't mean she doesn't have disordered eating. Second, athletes and coaches alike seem to believe that thin equals better performance, but they're wrong. *There is absolutely no evidence that low body weight or low body fat improves athletic performance.* Rather, it is being fit and healthy that allows optimal athletic performance, and no athlete can be optimally fit if she is underfueled.

Lastly, many female athletes have been reassured by coaches and even some doctors(!) that it's normal for athletes *not* to have a regular menstrual cycle, and that cessation of menstruation is just a normal consequence of training. From a health perspective, this is simply not acceptable. Lack of menstruation can be caused by many conditions other than the triad, including pregnancy, thyroid dysfunction, and anorexia. *Any time a woman's menstrual cycle is interrupted, there has to be a reason!* Cessation of menstruation should not be considered normal, because any time menses are interrupted, the female athlete is at risk for premature, possibly irreversible, osteoporosis. Therefore, any athlete who stops menstruating should be medically evaluated by a physician who is familiar with the female athlete triad and its potential for irreversible damage.

What should you do if you suspect that you, or someone you know, has the female athlete triad? Seek help from a health care team with experience treating the triad. Don't try to go it alone.

PART 5

WHAT EVERY ACTIVE WOMAN NEEDS TO KNOW ABOUT SPORTS INJURIES

<table>
<tr><td>

C
H
A
P
T
E
R
11

</td><td>

COMMON SPORTS INJURIES IN WOMEN

</td></tr>
</table>

Occasionally, a patient tells me she's afraid to exercise or try a sport because she's afraid of getting injured. True, injuries can be dramatic and heart-wrenching. We've all seen the anguished face of an athlete who one moment is at the top of her game and the next is on the ground, clutching an injury. Televised sports shows replay slow-motion footage of the injury occurring, and refer to injuries as "season-ending" and "dream-threatening." But rarely are athletic injuries life-threatening. Despite the drama, the truth is that most athletic injuries will heal in a matter of weeks to months, and the athlete will once again be back in top form, chasing her dreams. In contrast, the widespread medical illnesses common to women who don't exercise *are* life-threatening and, unfortunately, often permanent. Wouldn't we all rather risk an ankle sprain than a heart attack?

It's important to realize that injuries are an equal-opportunity fact of life. They happen now and then to everyone—exercisers and nonexercisers alike. The worst ankle sprain I've ever seen was in a woman who twisted her ankle stepping down from the curb, wearing four-inch stiletto heels. And I see more complaints of back pain in nonexercising women than in exercising ones, often due to lack of muscle strength and conditioning. So you shouldn't let fear of an injury keep you from getting all the health benefits of exercise. That said, it is important for you to know how to deal with an injury, should one occur. And more important, you should know what you can do to try to prevent an injury from ever occurring.

MOST SPORTS INJURIES ARE NOT GENDER RELATED

The media spotlight occasionally focuses on an injured female athlete, and inevitably, someone suggests that she got injured primarily because she's a woman. Recent research confirms that this is simply not true. Injury is more likely to be related to fitness level than gender. Both men and women who are out of shape are more likely to be injured than their more fit counterparts, regardless of gender.

Despite this welcome knowledge, there is a great deal that doctors still don't know about women's sports injuries. Unfortunately, because we have more questions than answers about some athletic injuries, there is no shortage of misinformation to fill in the missing pieces. This was underscored a few years ago, when a study published in a medical journal suggested that women are more likely to injure a particular knee ligament, the anterior cruciate ligament (ACL), because the ligament is sensitive to the effects of estrogen. This study was pounced upon by television and news journalists, and pretty soon, everyone was talking about the "hormone problem" that made women vulnerable to a potentially devastating athletic injury. Some time later, an astute researcher discovered flaws in the study that cast serious doubt on the accuracy of the study's results. But the damage was done: So many stories had been written with the initial information that it had already been accepted as fact in the sports community.

Occasionally, a modern-day naysayer reports that women are going to hurt themselves, particularly if they participate in a sport traditionally viewed as a man's sport, like football, hockey, or boxing. Like those of Victorian-era doctors, their views are based on personal, often unrecognized, bias. Although there is much we don't know, one of the things we're sure of is that the majority of sports injuries are sport-specific rather than gender-specific. Simply put, specific injuries are common in certain sports, and they occur in boys and girls, men and women. For instance, tennis elbow happens to both men and women tennis players; shoulder pain is common among both male and female swimmers; basketball players get a lot of sprained ankles.

Much of what has attracted the attention of the media, however, are a few injuries that affect girls and women more frequently than boys and men. Of course, it is very important that we learn to recognize these injury patterns so we can find ways to prevent them. But it is crucial that we keep the media spotlight in perspective. If we let attention to these topics start us down the slippery slope of thinking sports are dangerous for girls and women, we'll risk a return to the Victorian attitudes that women have worked so hard to overcome. I'll never forget one interview I had a few years ago with a television news producer. He wanted to produce a story about girls playing hockey, but it quickly became apparent that his bias was that hockey was "too dangerous" for girls. He did not have a shred of evidence to support his view, but he was firmly convinced that he was right. During our discussions, he eventually revealed that he thought it was unacceptable for girls to risk the cuts, bruises, broken bones, and lost teeth that can occur in hockey. When I asked him why it was acceptable for boys to risk such injuries but not girls, he responded, "Boys can go places in life with a few scars, but girls can't."

Are Women Different from Men?

Cosmetics aside, there are some real differences between the bodies of women and men, which begin to become apparent at puberty. Prior to puberty, boys and girls are roughly equal in size, speed, and growth. After the onset of puberty, girls have an increase in body fat, whereas body fat drops slightly in boys. Boys have a longer growth phase and higher levels of testosterone, so they generally end up bigger—taller and more muscular. Their bones usually continue growing until at least age twenty, whereas the average girl's bone growth is over a couple of years earlier. The resulting skeleton in women is made of thinner and lighter bones than the average man's, which is one of the main reasons women are more likely than men to develop osteoporosis.

Because of the differences in growth, the average adult female ends up about four or five inches shorter and thirty to forty pounds lighter than the average adult male. Many years ago, these anatomic differences were used as ammunition against women who wanted to play sports. Now we realize that these differences between men and women do not affect their respective abilities to play sports. In fact, there may be some advantages for the female athlete. Some researchers suspect that because a woman's build results in a slightly lower center of gravity, she may have a natural advantage in sports requiring good balance, like gymnastics and even soccer. Others believe that a woman's higher body fat percentage and smaller size allow her to exercise for a longer duration, which may ultimately prove to be an advantage in ultra-endurance sports.

A female skeleton also differs from a male skeleton by having a wider pelvis and narrower shoulders, which can result in different forces on the knee and elbow in women than in men. For instance, the wider pelvis (which allows for childbirth) means that the angle from the hip to the knee is larger in women than in men. Many sports medicine doctors believe this larger angle predisposes women to pain around the kneecap, a common condition known as *patellofemoral pain syndrome* (see page 265). And the typical woman's narrower shoulders means that she will have more of an angle at the elbow than the average man. This angle affects the way a woman throws a ball (hence, the scornful old expression "throwing like a girl"), and may also cause a tendency to lead with the elbow when playing a sport such as tennis. Such anatomical differences can be quite subtle, but they can have a tremendous effect on a girl or woman's athletic skills development. It is especially important for coaches working with female athletes to understand not just the specifics of their sport, but some of the specifics of working with female athletes. A coach aware of such anatomical differences understands that while this doesn't affect a woman's ability to excel at certain sports, it may affect equipment choices or training techniques.

COMMON SPORTS INJURIES

When most people think about athletic injuries, they envision an acute event, like an athlete twisting a knee or turning an ankle. While this type of acute, traumatic injury is dramatic, it is not the most common type of injury in active women. Rather, most injuries in active women are known as *overuse injuries*. Overuse injuries, as the name implies, means that an injury has occurred because of chronic wear and tear rather than an acute event. Overuse can occur to essentially any type of tissue in the human body, including muscle, tendons, and bones. *Tendinitis, bursitis,* and *fasciitis* are common overuse injuries to the body's soft tissues, whereas stress fractures are overuse injuries that affect the bone. Overuse injuries to both soft tissue and bone are common in women. In fact, data from the National Center for Health Statistics show that for men and women with musculoskeletal complaints, men are much more likely to report a specific injury to which they attribute their pain. Women, on the other hand, often do not report any injury that could have caused their discomfort. Many of them are suffering from an unrecognized overuse injury.

Overuse Injuries
Tendinitis

Muscles are attached to bone by thick bands of connective tissue called tendons. Whenever a muscle contracts, it tugs on its tendon, which is anchored to bone. In this chain, the tendon is a bit of a weak link, because it connects the powerful muscle with solid bone. When you use a muscle repetitively, injury can occur anywhere along the chain—to muscle, tendon, or bone—but most commonly affects the weakest link. When the vulnerable tendon becomes inflamed from repetitive use, the painful condition known as tendinitis results. Similarly, other structures like fascia (another type of connective tissue) and bursa (small protective pads near tendons) can also become inflamed from repetitive stress, causing conditions known respectively as fasciitis and bursitis.

In addition to pain, the inflammation (from Latin, it literally means "to set on fire") of a tendon, bursa, or fascia causes the affected tissue to swell and become warm and red. This inflammatory process is complex; once it's initiated, a tremendous variety of cells crowd into the injury site to offer input. Think about what happens when humans suffer a natural disaster: relief agencies, news reporters, and curious bystanders all flock to the scene. Some are very helpful; others block the roadways and generally just get in the way. That same type of response happens when a part of the body gets inflamed: some of the circulating cells supply crucial help to the injured tissue; others just create havoc. The longer the tissue stays inflamed, the more potential for lasting damage. Chronic inflammation can lead to scarring, atrophy, or permanent destruction of the tissue. If the problem becomes a chronic one, the obvious symptoms of inflammation subside, but only after the damage has been done. What's left behind is not unlike the scene of a house fire that has burned itself out: sometimes the remains are hardly recognizable. Doctors use the term *tendinosis* to describe tendons that have been damaged in this way.

Tendinitis is particularly common in the muscles we use frequently, including the hamstrings and calf muscles in the legs, and the rotator cuff and biceps in the shoulder. While tendinitis most commonly results from overuse, it can also be associated with seemingly unrelated medical conditions. In addition, pain in the muscles themselves, which can stem from a wide variety of conditions, can sometimes be misinterpreted as tendinitis. For example, I have seen muscle aches caused by everything from alcoholism to hypothyroidism blamed on tendinitis. Because tendinitis is so common, this is a mistake easily made by both doctors and their patients. So if you have what you think is recurrent tendinitis, or tendinitis affecting more than one area of your body, talk to your doctor about other diseases that could be masquerading as this common overuse injury.

Shin Splints

Shin splints is a popular term used to describe another very common overuse injury in the lower leg. Shin splints refers to pain along the edge of the tibia (the shinbone), where several of the muscles that control foot movement are attached. Instead of having a long, ropelike tendon, these muscles attach to bone by short, thick bands of fibrous tissue. Most doctors describe shin splints as inflammation of these muscular attachments, which occurs commonly in running and jumping sports, like track and field or basketball.

Several different factors contribute to development of shin splints, including muscle weakness and inflexibility. Pronating the foot (excessively rolling the foot inward) adds stress to the muscle attachments, increasing the likelihood of developing shin splints. This type of foot pronation seems to be especially common in women. Poorly fitting or worn-out shoes and exercising on hard surfaces often contributes to the development of shin splints. Some of my patients with mild shin splints have found that simply replacing old shoes with well-cushioned new ones and avoiding walking or running on concrete can eliminate the discomfort.

One of the most common misconceptions in sports medicine is that untreated shin splints become stress fractures. Not true! *These are two completely different injuries.* The confusion arises because both "shin splints" (i.e., soft tissue injuries) and stress fractures (i.e., bone injuries) commonly occur in the lower leg, or shin. I explain to patients that this is simply the medical equivalent of finding oranges (i.e., fruit) and broccoli (i.e., vegetables) in the produce section of the grocery store . . . they aren't related, they just happen to show up in the same area!

Stress Fractures

Many people tend to think of bone as a solid, rock-hard substance; in reality, bone is actually a very pliable living tissue. Viewed under a microscope, bone looks more like a sponge or a thick slice of Swiss cheese than a solid rock. Bone forms the human skeletal framework, anchoring our muscles and providing shelter for important organs like the brain and heart. And like the soft tissues of the body, bone is vulnerable to wear-and-tear type of injuries.

Bone serves as an important mineral "bank," where 98 percent of the body's calcium is stored. It is an extraordinarily busy bank, where deposits and withdrawals (of calcium) are constantly being made. Without this continual exchange, the many functions of the body that require calcium—like the beating of the heart—would cease. While the calcium is being shuttled in and out, the bone bank has special "workers" that scurry around, making sure every bone stays dense and strong. When they find an area that needs some repair work, they recruit other cells to help complete the job. Bone is undergoing this process, called "remodeling and repair," twenty-four hours a day.

Exercise stimulates these remodeling and repair crews, encouraging them to make the bones even stronger. But too much exercise can overwhelm these hard workers, and they reach a point at which they simply can't keep up with the demands for repair. When this happens, tiny cracks, or *stress fractures,* appear in the bone.

Stress fractures can occur in any bone in the body, but they are most common in the legs and feet. They initially cause pain only with activity, like walking or running, but may eventually cause constant pain, even while sleeping. Most will heal within a few weeks, if rested. Ignored, however, a stress fracture can progress to a completely broken bone, requiring surgical repair, turning an overuse injury into a much more serious one.

Although stress fractures occur in both men and women, they are more common in women. This was first noticed among military recruits, where women were found to be developing stress fractures up to twelve times more frequently than men. Several studies suggested that stress fractures were most common in the female recruits who were the least physically fit at the beginning of their military training. Female athletes, especially runners, also seem to be more susceptible to stress fractures, although at much lower rates than their military counterparts.

Why do women seem to be more susceptible to this type of bone injury? No one knows for sure. Some experts believe that it is simply the fact that women have smaller, less dense bones than do men. Others believe it is related to differences in biomechanics (referring to the way we move). And in young women who overexercise, have unhealthy diets, and lose their menstrual period, stress fractures are often the first sign of a syndrome known as the female athlete triad (see page 247).

Kneecap Pain

The single most common injury I see in women is an overuse syndrome with many different names, including *patellofemoral pain syndrome, chondromalacia, runner's knee,* and *anterior knee pain.* It is an equal opportunity injury: it also affects women who don't exercise. It crosses the boundary between a soft tissue overuse injury and bone injury, because kneecap pain can come from the soft tissues around the kneecap or from the kneecap itself. Women who have this problem often have pain that not only affects their ability to exercise but interferes with everyday life. The pain is frequently constant and gets worse with any activity. Going up, and especially down, stairs makes the pain worse. It even worsens with prolonged sitting—such as at a movie or desk, and during car or airplane travel. Doctors sometimes call this the "movie" or "theater" sign.

Why does this happen? The kneecap, or *patella* (a Latin term meaning "little plate"), is a small bone that is actually embedded in the tendon of the quadriceps (anterior thigh) muscle. Whenever you use the quadriceps muscle to straighten your knee, the patella glides up and down with the muscle and its tendon. It also tilts and rotates a bit, helping your quadriceps get the most power out of every contraction. The patella glides along a smooth track created by an indentation in the end of the thighbone (*femur*). If the patella is forced to move off this smooth track, the whole knee suffers. Think of the patella like a train: if a train jumps off its track, pandemonium occurs. Unfortunately, a woman's anatomy seems to be predisposed to this occurrence. Look at the typical man: his knees line up pretty much under his hips, in a straight line, which helps the patella stay in its track at the end of the thighbone. But the typical woman has a wider pelvis, so her hips line up outside her knees. The end result is that the patella tends to slip off its track more easily, causing pain.

This condition can occur in anyone, but it's especially common in women whose hip and quadriceps muscles are weak or inflexible. The *quadriceps* (Latin for "four heads") muscle is actually a group of four muscles. The weaker the quadriceps, the easier it is for the patella to slip off its track. This is especially true if the inner one of the four quadriceps muscles (known as the *vastus medialis obliquus,* or VMO) is weak. Additionally, weak muscles around the hip seem to lead to overburdening of the knee, adding to the woes of the patella.

And as with other overuse injuries, foot pronation, exercising on a hard surface, or simply doing too much can contribute to pain around the patella. Even wearing high heels can cause it! Of all the athletic patients I see with this condition, the ones most commonly affected are runners and devotees of step aerobics. This is not surprising, because both activities are impact ones that require repetitive bending and straightening the knee.

Occasionally, I see a patient with kneecap pain who has been told that she should just stop exercising. Because of the many health benefits of exercise, I never think this is a good answer. Besides, this injury is common in women whether they exercise or not. Instead, I recommend figuring out why she was susceptible to the injury and correcting the causes.

Many athletic women with kneecap pain have gotten relief by taping their kneecaps, or by wearing a brace or small strap designed to help control patella motion. If the primary cause of pain is a weak quadriceps muscle, wearing a brace that helps keep the patella properly aligned can be helpful. This can be a simple pull-on elastic sleeve with a hole cut out for the kneecap, available in most drugstores, or a more sophisticated one prescribed by a sports medicine doctor. But I always remind my patients that a brace is meant to be a temporary solution. Addressing the underlying problem, whether by strengthening weak muscles, altering exercise habits, or getting new shoes, is ultimately the smartest move.

TIPS FOR AVOIDING KNEE PAIN

Do:

Avoid high heels (two inches or more) as much as possible.

Stretch and strengthen the quadriceps and hip muscles.

Cross-train by biking.

Don't:

Wear worn-out athletic shoes.

Rely on a brace without addressing the cause.

Try to exercise through pain.

Acute Injuries

Accidents happen. Sometimes, even when you're doing everything right, you get injured. An oncoming cyclist veers her bike into yours; you grab a rebound and turn your ankle when you land on another basketball player's foot; you collide with the catcher at home plate. In an athletic setting, the most common acute injuries in women are *sprains,* which are injuries to ligaments, and *strains,* which are injuries to muscles or tendons. You may be surprised to know that in adults, such soft tissue injuries are much more common than fractures, but in children, the reverse is true.

Sprains

Ligaments are thick bands of fibrous tissue that connect bones to each other. There are hundreds of ligaments throughout the body, connecting bones in joints. Ligaments function in a very important way: They help stabilize joints by allowing normal range of motion, while preventing excessive motion. Ligaments are frequently injured when a joint is forced beyond its normal range of motion. For instance, "twisting" an ankle causes stretching of the ankle ligaments; if it is twisted too far, the ligaments can tear. When an injured patient tells me she heard or felt a pop, I know she probably has a torn ligament. When ligaments are injured, the joint can become too mobile, or unstable.

Injuries to ligaments are typically graded from first to third degree, according to the extent of injury. First-degree sprains are ones in which the ligament fibers have been stretched but not torn. Although the injury is painful, the joint's stability is not jeopardized. In second-degree sprains the ligament has been partially torn, while third degree indicates a complete tear. As the degree of injury rises, the risk of instability of the joint increases as well.

Women and ACL Injuries

For unclear reasons, women generally tend to have more joint laxity (looseness) than men do. Research has shown that ligaments are influenced by a variety of factors, including the presence of estrogen. It is commonly believed that estrogen makes ligaments more supple, but whether this is an advantage, disadvantage, or neither remains to be seen. In general, women are not thought to have substantially more ligament injuries than men. One of the most highly publicized exceptions is injury to the anterior cruciate ligament, or ACL, in the knee.

The ACL is one of four main ligaments that provides knee stability. It helps keep the knee "centered" by preventing the tibia (shinbone) from shifting forward. Female athletes, particularly those who participate in soccer and basketball, seem to tear this ligament up to eight times more frequently than their male counterparts. At the time of this writing, we still don't know why. Some researchers believe that the fluctuation of estrogen with the menstrual cycle is the culprit behind the increased number of injuries. But since estrogen affects not just one, but all of the hundreds of ligaments in our bodies, this theory never made much sense to me. Why would this increase only the risk of ACL injuries, and not all other ligament injuries?

Recently, promising research has focused on differences in the ways female athletes move and "recruit" muscles.

Watch a group of women play basketball—and then watch a group of men play. Women tend to land from a jump, such as rebounding a basketball, on a straight (not bent) knee, and on one leg rather than two. Men, on the other hand, are more likely to land in a crouched position. Also, studies have shown us that women tend to rely heavily on the quadriceps muscle in the front of the thigh, and that they have weaker and less responsive hamstrings in the back of the thigh. The quadriceps muscle is primarily responsible for straightening the knee, while the hamstring bends the knee. If the stronger quadriceps overpowers the hamstring, the knee can be overstraightened, or hyperextended, resulting in a torn ACL.

Is there anything you can do to decrease your own risk of an ACL injury? I think so. Some researchers have trained female athletes to change their patterns of movement, resulting in a decrease in the expected number of ACL injuries. The Cincinnati Sports Medicine and Research Foundation has produced a videotape of such training tips that is available to the public. You can also check with the sports medicine experts in your area for workshops and seminars that teach these techniques.

Strains

As a group, muscle and tendon strains are probably the single most common acute injury. Just like with ligament sprains, a muscle strain is usually graded by degree of injury, from stretching to complete tear. A strain can occur in the muscle itself, or in its tendon. Many people believe that lack of flexibility is the greatest cause of muscle strains.

Muscles are anchored by a tendon to one bone, and reach across a joint to attach by another tendon to another bone. When a muscle contracts, it shortens, pulling the two bones toward each other and creating joint movement. Even though we all use our muscles in this way thousands of times each day, most of us never give any thought to how they work. But every movement requires the coordinated effort of several muscles, known as *agonists* and *antagonists*. All the muscles that produce movement in one direction are agonists, whereas those creating movement in the opposite direction are antagonists. For instance, when you use the biceps to bend your elbow, bringing your hand toward your head, several smaller muscles (agonists) also contract and help guide your hand exactly where you want it to go. While these muscles are contracting, the triceps (antagonist) relaxes and stretches. When you are ready to straighten your elbow, the process reverses: the triceps shortens by contracting, and the biceps lengthens by relaxing. Without these muscle pairs, many basic activities that we take for granted, like eating, would be impossible.

A muscle strain is likely when a forceful contraction occurs while the muscle is in a stretched (lengthened) position. For instance, when a sprinter is racing, the hamstring muscle is rapidly contracting and relaxing as she is propelled forward. When her leg is stretched out ahead, the hamstring is in its lengthened position. To continue moving forward, she must quickly bring that foot to the ground, forcefully contracting the hamstring. Timing is crucial; if she contracts the hamstring while it is still stretched, the force may actually cause the muscle to tear. While this can happen to any muscle, muscles that cross two joints or have more fast twitch fibers, like the hamstring and *gastrocnemius* (calf muscle), are especially vulnerable.

MUSCLE CRAMPS

Muscle cramps are essentially spasms that occur when the normal cycle of muscle contraction and relaxation is interrupted. Despite their common occurrence, cramps are a bit of a mystery. We know they can occur for a variety of reasons, including overexertion, dehydration, poor conditioning, or an imbalance of *electrolytes,* including sodium and potassium. Since the presence of calcium is also required for muscle contraction, inadequate calcium intake may also be a cause of muscle cramps. If you're experiencing muscle cramps, try increasing your fluid intake. Eat more potassium-rich foods (such as bananas), and be sure your calcium intake is adequate. If you're low on sodium, you're probably going to know it, because you'll be craving salty foods. Don't be afraid to use the salt shaker, but skip the salt tablets. Most of us already get several times more salt than we need, and dumping several hundred milligrams of salt in the form of a pill into your stomach might just make you feel ill. Worse, too much salt makes you excrete extra calcium, a nutrient most women can't afford to lose! And remember, cramps may have nothing to do with your nutritional state. Anecdotally, some supplements like creatine have been associated with cramping. Don't forget to stretch, and if the cramps continue, consult your doctor.

Just like with a ligament sprain, a muscle strain may be heralded by a pop. Depending on the degree of injury, there may be swelling and a lump (formed by a torn muscle, or by a collection of blood known as a *hematoma*). You may notice bruising, which doctors call *ecchymosis,* which also indicates bleeding from the torn tissue. If the muscle is completely torn, you may not be able to contract it at all, meaning you will have difficulty performing the movements that muscle is responsible for. Remember, most muscles have several

MASSAGE

Stand right past the finish line of any marathon, and you're likely to be trampled by racers making a beeline for the massage tent. Elite-level athletes, weekend warriors, and gym rats all swear by their postexercise massage habits. But other than making a tired body feel good, does massage really work?

The jury's still out. Many massage therapists continue to assert that a postexercise rubdown rids the muscles of lactic acid, a by-product of exercise, and stimulates oxygen delivery to the tired muscles. So far, though, no reliable research has shown this to be true. There is also no evidence that massage improves performance or prevents injuries. And a bad massage could actually be detrimental. It does seem, however, that massage can help improve muscle flexibility and tone and decrease delayed-onset muscle soreness. Before you plunk down the typical $50-plus fee, do a little research to help you decide whether you're interested in Swedish massage (the grandmother of massage techniques, it spawned the back rub that many women associate with massage), a sports massage (which is typically deep and vigorous and may focus on especially tight muscles), or one of the other many contemporary interpretations of massage. Look for a licensed massage therapist who has experience working with athletes. And remember, no massage is a substitute for stretching and proper training!

helpers (agonists), so even if you have torn one muscle you may still be able to move the joint.

One mistake that's commonly made by my patients who've injured a muscle is the tendency to test the injury. Too many people are tempted to try exercising to see how bad it really is. Talk about adding insult to injury! Injured athletes—particularly the "weekend warriors"—seem to have a compulsion to do this, repetitively contracting and relaxing a muscle to see how much it hurts. It reminds me of a child who can't resist sticking her finger in a small hole in her sock, turning a small hole into a large one. If you have a small muscle tear and you can't resist testing it, you will probably succeed in making the tear bigger. Resist the urge to test your injury and get an ice pack on it as soon as you can. And if you heard, or felt, a distinct pop, see a doctor.

CHAPTER 12

AVOIDING INJURY

MANY OVERUSE INJURIES, and even some traumatic ones, are pre-
ventable. How can you prevent getting injured? A number of
factors, including shoes and equipment, training habits, and
underlying muscle imbalances can contribute to the development of an injury. Finding such predisposing factors for
the injury is just as important as diagnosing and treating it,
so the athlete can prevent it from occurring again. A good
sports medicine doctor plays detective, tracking down clues
to the cause of injury. You can learn how to do this, too,
so you can spot the risk factors in your own exercise program . . . before you get injured!

MAKING SMART TRAINING CHOICES

Alice, a forty-one-year-old hospital administrator, came into my office complaining of heel and ankle pain. She had been running intermittently for several years, but since getting a promotion a year ago, she had found herself too busy to exercise. Frustrated because she had gained fifteen pounds, she committed to running every morning. After a couple of months, she began having the pain that brought her into my office.

Alice was suffering from Achilles tendinitis, a common injury in runners. It wasn't hard to diagnose or treat her injury; the challenge was finding where she had gone wrong so she could prevent the same mistakes in the future. Alice made her first mistake when she resumed running every day. Although she was familiar with the fitness factors of intensity, duration, and frequency, she thought that they didn't apply to her because she wasn't a novice exerciser. She was amazed when I told her that her body had lost essentially all of the benefits of years of exercise after several months of inactivity. She needed to start all over, just as if she was a beginner who had never exercised. And she had forgotten that rest days are important for everyone, from the most novice exerciser to the most elite. Rest days allow the body's repair process the time and energy to fix any microdamage to muscles, tendons, bones, and ligaments. And, as we age, our bodies often need a little longer to recover from exercise. Because Alice was exercising every day, her body's repair process never got a chance to complete its job.

Because Alice felt so pressed for time, she made another common mistake: she neglected to stretch. While stretching hasn't been proven to prevent injuries, most runners find it eases muscle tightness and its associated aches and pains.

Many sports medicine doctors think that stretching reduces the chance of muscle strain. Stretching the calf muscles and Achilles tendon is especially important in women like Alice, who wear high heels all day. High heels eventually lead to shortening and tightening of the tendon, which can be offset by gentle stretching.

Alice was in good company. Like over half of my patients, she had fallen into the trap that, in my experience, is the single most common cause of injury: the "too much, too soon, too fast" trap. Most women can stay out of this trap and cut their risk of injury in half by following the 10 to 15 percent progression rule. Progress your exercise program by choosing just one fitness factor, like duration, and increase it by *no more than* 10 to 15 percent each week. For instance, if you've begun a walking program by walking twenty minutes three or four days each week, progress weekly by increasing the time spent on each walk by two or three minutes. Within four weeks you will have gradually gotten to thirty minutes. At that point, choose to either keep increasing your duration of exercise, or add an extra day of exercise. While you may have to start off slower than you'd planned, following the 10 to 15 percent progression rule will get you wherever you're going, while minimizing your risk of injury. I remind patients who are impatient to progress of the fable of the slow but sure tortoise who wins out over the shortsighted hare!

DON'T IGNORE YOUR WEAKNESSES

Let's face it, we all have a tendency to play to our strengths. And while that may help you get ahead at the office, when it comes to exercise, it will put you on the track to injury. Why? Because our bodies are like complex machines—and every part serves an important purpose. Let's go back again to the analogy of a car. Let's say that you faithfully get engine tune-ups and oil changes, but that you neglect the tires. You won't realize that the tread has worn off one of your tires until it suddenly blows out on the road. You'd feel silly looking back and saying, "But look at all the times I changed the oil," because you realize that did nothing to prevent the tires from failing.

Our bodies are like that, too. They are more than just the sum of many parts; each part works together with the rest to keep us strong, energetic, and healthy. So exercising one part—like the heart, through cardiovascular exercises—while ignoring strength training and stretching means you only end up with a strong "engine." While that's very important, it doesn't do you much good if your skeleton's bones and muscles are too weak to get you where you're going.

Many women who do strength train choose to work on one part of their bodies and ignore the rest. Too many women are still thinking about the cosmetic benefits they'll gain, rather than the functional payoff of exercise. Frequently, they choose to exercise a muscle in the front of the body that they can see—like the biceps in the arm or the quadriceps in the front of the thigh—and ignore the corresponding muscle—like the triceps or hamstrings—on the back of the body. This sort of "out of sight, out of mind" thinking causes development of muscle imbalances, which can also lead to injury. Remember that muscles come in pairs called agonists and antagonists (see page 271). Exercising one without the other creates a strength imbalance, which can lead to injury.

Back pain, one of the most common complaints among women (whether they exercise or not), is often the result of such muscle imbalances. The so-called core muscles in the back and abdomen are an extremely important agonist-antagonist group of muscles. In addition to playing a critical role in maintaining good posture, they assist in a wide variety of movements, including kicking a ball, swinging a tennis racket, and lifting (weights, children, packages, etc.). Many women think that by doing sit-ups, they are taking care of the core muscles—but they're wrong. While sit-ups help strengthen one of the abdominal muscles, the rectus abdominus, they don't do much for the three other abdominal muscles, or for the very important muscles in the back. Paying attention to *all* of these muscles can help reduce the risk of back pain and injury.

Even weak muscles do their best to keep working. Because there are over 600 muscles in the body, a weak muscle can try to recruit others to help it do its job. If a big, important muscle is weak, many of the smaller ones around it try to pitch in. But when a small muscle answers the call for help from a larger muscle, it becomes vulnerable to injury, too. (Think of what would happen if a child tries to do an adult's job . . . sooner or later, there will be some big problems!) The end result? You end up with not one but multiple injuries to heal!

How Do You Spot Your Own Weaknesses?

Take a good, honest look at your exercise routine. Are there types of exercises, like stretching, that you avoid? Are there certain muscles you pay attention to but others you neglect? Do you notice differences in strength or flexibility between your right and left sides? Chances are good that without even realizing it, you've been ignoring your own "weak link," which leaves you vulnerable to an overuse injury. Once you recognize where your vulnerabilities are, adjust your exercise plan to correct them. Some of the weaknesses my patients frequently identify include:

- Avoiding strength training for the legs. This is a common error of many exercisers, especially runners and walkers. They tend to think that because they run, or walk, their legs are strong. Not necessarily true! Their legs have developed endurance but not muscle strength. Strong legs are the platform for many of our daily activities, including climbing stairs and bending and lifting. Weak legs mean our arms and back must do more work, which leaves them vulnerable to injury as well.

- Avoiding strength training for the upper body. Women tend to have weaker arms than legs, which is a good reason to work on strength training the upper body. Paradoxically, many women just choose to ignore their weaker muscles. But sitting at a computer for hours, putting groceries away, or carrying a child strains the weak muscles on a daily basis, so that any additional stress can cause the weak link to crumble. This is often the case with women who come in complaining of shoulder pain after just one leisurely weekend game of tennis. The tennis game was the proverbial straw that broke the camel's back: the real culprit was the underlying lack of muscle strength and conditioning.

- Skipping stretching. Many of my busy patients find time to squeeze in an exercise session, like twenty minutes on the treadmill, but they don't feel they have time to stretch. My routine suggestion is that, of the twenty minutes they have for exercise, eighteen can be spent on the treadmill, with two minutes left for stretching the calves, hamstrings, and quadriceps. This simple solution is generally met by hesitation. Many women frankly admit that they want to spend every minute they can in calorie-burning exercise, rather than "wasting time" stretching. But since stretching improves joint range of motion (allowing smoother, faster movements) and has been shown to help muscles become stronger, that two-minute commitment can actually help you burn more calories. And while stretching hasn't clearly been proven to prevent injuries, an overwhelming majority of the runners and walkers I see with overuse injuries like tendinitis and shin splints are the very ones who have avoided stretching.

- Skipping the warm-up phase. At the beginning of an exercise session or athletic event, spending just five to ten minutes warming up may help to prevent muscle strains. There is nothing magic about a warm-up; you don't have to do any special exercises in any special order. The idea is just to begin increasing your heart rate by walking briskly, swinging your arms, jogging in place, or slowly pedaling a bike. This type of warming up serves to increase blood flow to the large muscles you'll be using for exercise. This extra blood flow increases the muscle's temperature, making it warm. Warm muscles are more pliable, so they are able to easily contract and lengthen as needed, decreasing the risk of a strain. I have seen too many women hurry onto the tennis court without warming up, and end up in my office with a calf strain.

- Inadequate rehabilitation from a former injury. It's not uncommon that we forget we had an injury as soon as it doesn't hurt anymore. But just because the pain has subsided doesn't necessarily mean the injury has healed. Taking the time to rehabilitate the injury by improving weaknesses in strength, flexibility, and balance is one of the most important ways you can prevent injury recurrence. Lydia, a college basketball player, wishes she had realized the importance of rehabilitation after her first ankle sprain. Because she never rehabilitated her ankle after the first sprain, she was left with a weaker, less stable ankle, which she continued to reinjure in several games. During her last game, she not only reinjured the old sprain, she tore another ligament, too. At this point, rehabilitation is no longer enough: Lydia's injury requires surgery.

- Settling for inadequate gear. Now that we recognize some of the physical variations (like shorter and lighter skeletons, and increased angles at the knees and elbows) that can affect women's sports performance, we realize how important it is for women to have gear that fits. The importance of choosing the right shoes and other equipment can't be overemphasized, because a poor fit can lead to injury.

WARNING SIGNS OF IMPENDING INJURY

You know how the television weatherman uses a storm-tracking system to alert you to the development and approach of hurricanes? Your body has a similar surprisingly good system for alerting you to the first signs of injury. But many of us have unconsciously gotten good at ignoring those signals. How can you learn to spot the warnings? It's as simple as learning to listen to your body. First, pay attention to fatigue. Are you simply tired from a difficult day or too little sleep? Are you hungry or thirsty? Or have you been exercising too hard or too frequently? If you feel tired at the beginning of your workout, either shorten the duration or lighten the intensity of your planned exercise session. If your feeling of fatigue is persistent, talk to your doctor about other possible causes. Ignoring the fatigue factor can cause your form to suffer, leaving you prone to mistakes and injury.

The fatigue factor also contributes to acute, traumatic injuries. Watch sporting events closely, and you'll notice that many injuries don't occur during the first part of a game, but rather later, when participants are getting tired.

EXERCISE IN THE HEAT

Your ability to tolerate heat depends on a variety of factors, including your size, age, and fitness level. Generally, high temperatures are harder to tolerate if you're very young or very old, have excess body fat, or have a low level of fitness. Not getting enough water, carbohydrates, and sleep can also make it harder for you to tolerate exercise in the heat.

If you're planning to exercise in a hot or humid environment, try to *acclimate* slowly. Start slowly and for shorter periods of time, and gradually increase only one of the fitness factors, like intensity or duration, at a time. Expect to sweat a lot, and be sure to drink plenty of fluids. Wear lightweight, light-colored clothing, preferably made from a good wicking material. Learn to recognize the warning signs of overheating, including nausea, dizziness, confusion, headache, and muscle cramps. If you experience any of these, stop exercise *immediately,* seek the shade, cool off, and rehydrate. Ignoring the early signs of heat stress can leave you at risk for heatstroke, a life-threatening condition that can come upon you rapidly.

EXERCISE IN THE COLD

Just as with exercise in the heat, how well you tolerate exercise in the cold depends on a variety of factors, including body size, body fat, and muscle mass. This is where your weight training program can really pay off, because metabolically active muscle generates lots of heat, keeping you warmer during cold weather activities. Extra body fat also provides insulation, but it isn't as efficient at keeping you warm as extra muscle mass is.

The more fit you are, the better you'll be able to tolerate exercise in the cold. Remember to warm up a little longer, and don't forget to stretch. It's also important that you dress appropriately: wear layers, with the bottom layer made of a wicking material (not cotton, which will trap sweat next to your body and cause chilling). Don't forget that you lose a lot of heat from your head, so a hat is very important. Add gloves or mittens, and an outer layer that is wind- and water-repellent.

Similarly, the majority of patients I see who've injured their knees skiing do so during one of the last runs of the day. So often, a woman who is hobbling in on crutches will say, "I knew I was getting tired, but my friends talked me into one more run." When your body is fatigued, your muscles can't respond to commands as quickly or completely, and your reaction time is slowed, both common causes of injury.

And forget about "no pain, no gain." Although a challenging workout might leave you feeling exhausted and a bit sore, pain is never a good thing, and it's not a normal consequence of exercise. If you feel pain during exercise, don't try to "walk it off." Stop and see if you can figure out what's causing your discomfort. Are you wearing new shoes (or, alternatively, a pair that's worn out)? Did you run more hills than usual, try a new machine at the gym, or exercise with a new partner? Invariably, when I ask a patient about changes in her routine, the knee-jerk response is "no changes," but as our conversation continues, she frequently remembers otherwise. If you stop and assess your situation, chances are you can figure out what went wrong. Try to exercise through pain, however, and you're much more likely to end up visiting someone like me—a sports medicine doctor.

TREATING AN INJURY

ALTHOUGH GENERALLY women are more likely than men to make visits to physicians, this does not seem to hold true in the area of sports medicine. I have encountered many women who try to ignore an injury for as long as possible. It is not uncommon for a woman to wait months, or even years, before coming in to have an injury, or pain, evaluated. Although there are often many reasons for the delay, there is one explanation that I have heard repeatedly from women, but that I have rarely heard from men: Women are afraid that they will simply be told to stop exercise. There are two reasons a woman seems to expect—and fear—this response. The first is that exercise has become an extremely important part of her self-identity, but she doesn't feel that she'll be taken seriously as an athlete. The second is common among women who use exercise for weight control: many would rather exercise through pain than stop and risk gaining weight.

However, the longer the injury has been around, the worse it tends to become, necessitating a longer recovery period. But that doesn't mean giving up all exercise. One of the first things I tell patients is that because of its many benefits, I almost never recommend that a woman *stop* exercise, although she will probably need to *modify* her exercise program while we treat her injury. For example, a runner with shin splints or a stress fracture can often still swim, ride a stationary bike, and work on strength training for the upper body. A swimmer with a shoulder injury can switch to a stair stepper or stationary bike, and work on strength training for the legs and core (abdomen and lower back) muscles. Being injured doesn't have to be synonymous with being inactive!

RICE

Occasionally, an athletic injury results in a tear, fracture, or dislocation that requires surgical repair. Many injuries, however, can be treated *conservatively,* a term doctors use to mean "without surgery." Whether your injury ultimately requires surgery may in part be determined not be your doctor, but by *your* initial response to injury. Almost everyone has heard the acronym RICE applied to first aid for sports injuries, but judging from the patients in my office, not everyone knows what it means.

Here, a brief review:

- R is for REST. Don't try to walk it off and continue exercising! Even if you think the injury is minor, take a break from exercise. I have never seen anyone who is sorry that she took this simple precaution, but I have seen a lot of injured people who were unhappy that they didn't! Wait twenty-four to forty-eight hours, and if you remain pain-free, consider that the green light to resume exercise. Not infrequently, patients admit that a severe injury was preceded by a minor one that was ignored.

- I is for ICE. Ice is nature's own anti-inflammatory. Whether from overuse or a traumatic mishap, all injuries go through the process of inflammation, during which cells in the injured area release a variety of chemicals and hormones. The inflammatory process begins immediately when an injury occurs, and is actually responsible for much of the pain, swelling, and disability that accompanies an injury. Because of this, the first line of treatment for an injury traditionally involves anti-inflammatory measures, and nothing is safer or more effective than properly applied ice. Apply the ice for twenty minutes out of every hour for a few hours. And remember that more is not better! Leaving an ice pack on for more than twenty minutes raises the risk of freezing the skin and other tissues. Just because ice is natural doesn't mean it can't cause harm if not used appropriately.

- C is for COMPRESSION. Many people skip this step, but it is extremely effective. Using an Ace bandage, wrap the injured area securely, but not too tightly. (If the area below your bandage takes on a bluish hue or feels numb, loosen the bandage.) Providing some pressure can help reduce swelling, which can help lessen recovery time.

- E is for ELEVATION. Gravity alone contributes to swelling, so elevating the injured area negates this unwanted effect. Remember, you must elevate the injured area above the level of your heart for maximum benefit. This often means lying down, with your injury propped up on a pillow.

There are two alternate acronyms to RICE, PRICE and RICES. Both the P (for protection) and the S (for support) refer to the concept of using devices such as crutches, slings, or splints to help support and protect the injured area, both of which are usually a good idea.

HEAT OR ICE?

Ice is nature's own anti-inflammatory: it helps to limit swelling as well as pain. For seventy-two hours after an acute injury, choose ice over heat; while heat may initially feel good, it causes dilation of the blood vessels, increasing circulation to the site of injury, which may result in more swelling. Ice for fifteen minutes out of each hour you can, ideally several times a day. Don't apply ice directly to the skin (you can cause a nasty burn this way!), and never fall asleep with an ice pack in place.

Quick tip: A bag of frozen vegetables makes a terrific low-fuss, low-mess ice pack. Just use it as though it were a bag of crushed ice, and refreeze after each use. (You may want to label one bag in your freezer as the designated ice pack or the finicky eaters in the family may have a new excuse not to eat their veggies!)

ASSISTING THE HEALING PROCESS

Hopefully, you followed the RICE principles, limiting the extent of the injury. Now, what can you do to aid the actual healing process?

Dealing with Inflammation

Many people run to their medicine cabinets and grab a bottle of medication. But wait! Don't take that pill until you really understand how it might help—or hurt—you. During the inflammatory process, one of the chemicals released is known as *prostaglandins*. Common medications, including aspirin, ibuprofen, and naproxen, are known as anti-inflammatory medications because they block the production of prostaglandins. This, in turn, helps to reduce pain and swelling, which can decrease injury recovery time. But there is some concern that reducing prostaglandins creates an open field for other, potentially more harmful chemicals to wreak havoc. Additionally, anti-inflammatory medications are not without side effects. They can cause stomach upsets, allergic reactions, ulcers, and kidney and liver problems. And because of potential for damage to the fetus, they should be avoided during pregnancy.

How do you decide whether or not to use such a common medication? In general, if you are otherwise healthy and have a lot of pain and swelling, the pros of anti-inflammatory medications probably outweigh the cons. Depending on the degree of injury, your doctor may recommend a prescription-strength anti-inflammatory medication, or may even recommend an injection of *cortisone,* the most potent of anti-inflammatories. If, however, you have mild pain without significant swelling, consider using a medication like *acetaminophen* (e.g., Tylenol) that works to decrease pain but has no effect on the inflammatory process. And remember that ice, nature's own anti-inflammatory, is an option for managing both pain and swelling.

Although inflammation is a painful process, it serves an important purpose. In addition to heralding the arrival of the body's "repairmen," it alerts you to the fact that an injury has occurred and encourages you to stop using the injured area so that healing can begin. It's important to realize that using ice or taking anti-inflammatory medications will help you feel better but won't help your injury heal, which is why treating pain is only the first small step in treating a sports injury. If, in fact, you use medications so that you can continue exercising while ignoring the injury, you are increasing the chance that your injury will worsen!

Whether or not you choose to actively treat the inflammation, it will eventually resolve, because no tissue can stay

---

CORTISONE: THE MAGIC BULLET?

Watch any major sports event, and you're likely to hear about an athlete getting an injection of cortisone. Although informally called a steroid, cortisone is very different than the anabolic steroids used by some athletes and bodybuilders. Cortisone is in a class of steroids known as *corticosteroids,* and is a very potent anti-inflammatory medication. Cortisone can be given by pill or injection. It is generally used to treat chronic inflammatory processes, like arthritis and bursitis. Although cortisone can provide dramatic reduction in inflammation, it can also cause the injected tissue to weaken or rupture, and can increase the risk of infection. Because of these potentially severe side effects, it is not usually used for acute sports injuries.

---

inflamed forever. Either way, the injured tissue has the potential to eventually heal. Just like a house that has been burned down can be built back up again, tissues that have been damaged by inflammation can be reconstructed, a process that doctors refer to as *remodeling.* But this healing process requires time. Many times, an athlete's recovery from an injury is prolonged because she keeps testing it before it has completely healed. I tell my patients that this is like building part of the burned house again, and then tearing it down before construction is completed.

The Role of Physical Therapy

In my opinion, physical therapy is one of the best treatment approaches for most sports injuries, with one caveat: You must be under the tutelage of a good therapist. Too often, a patient who comes to me for a second opinion says that she tried physical therapy, but it didn't work. When I ask what treatment she had, there is usually a list that goes something like this: ice, ultrasound, massage, and stretching. Most patients who get better with this passive treatment would have gotten better simply with the passage of time. Of course, there is nothing wrong with using the techniques called *modalities,* like ultrasound and electrical stimulation, but they are the icing on the cake. The mainstay of physical therapy is *exercise therapy.*

After evaluating your injury, a good physical therapist will recommend appropriate exercises for correcting deficiencies in a variety of areas, like strength, flexibility, balance, and posture. In addition to the sessions spent with the therapist, you should be given a "prescription" for exercises to do at home. Do them. No matter how busy you are. How quickly your injury resolves and you get back to doing your regular activities is largely in *your own* hands. When I refer patients to physical therapy, I ask them to return to the office in a few weeks. Invariably, the ones who are happiest with their progress are the ones who have faithfully done their home exercise program.

Some tips for finding a good physical therapist:

- Look for a therapist trained in sports medicine. Just like doctors, physical therapists often specialize, so one who worked well with your cousin's spine injury may not be the right one for your tennis elbow. For example, if you have a foot injury, seek out a therapist who works with runners or dancers; a shoulder injury, search for one with experience treating swimmers or pitchers.
- Ask about credentials and experience. A well-qualified therapist is happy to tell you about his or her training.
- Shop around. Ask for recommendations from your doctor, local sports medicine clinics, or health clubs.

Don't Stop Eating

I have seen too many women make the mistake of cutting back on the amount they eat when they become injured. One of the most important ways you can assist injury healing is by providing the nutritional building blocks needed for tissue repair. But many women, worried that they will gain weight with decreased activity, severely restrict their diets, limiting the injured tissue's access to the very tools it needs for repair and recovery. In addition to their usual functions, nutrients play a special role in the healing process. Strive for well-balanced meals, paying special attention to the following:

- Carbohydrates, which provide energy for healing.
- Protein, which is used to repair damaged tissue; if carbohydrates aren't available for energy, protein will be diverted from the repair process and used as an energy source instead.
- Fats, which provide energy and are the building blocks for several hormones and the immune system.
- Calcium, important for building bone, is also needed for muscles to function.
- Iron, which transports oxygen to the injured tissue.
- Zinc and vitamins A, C, and K aid some of the chemical reactions required for tissue repair.
- Water, which gets used in the tissue repair process.

GETTING BACK IN THE GAME

One of the first questions an injured athlete wants to have answered is: How long before I can play again? Because of individual variables, that is an impossible question to answer with precision. The speed with which an injury heals is influenced by several factors, including the athlete's compliance with the prescribed treatment, such as rest and rehabilitation, as well as appropriate nutrition. Patience is an injured athlete's best friend, because trying to get back in the game too soon is one of the most frequent causes of reinjury.

If you had an injury that you've managed with the RICE principle and you're ready to play again, ask yourself the following questions:

Has the pain disappeared?
Is range of motion normal?
Do you think you could recognize warning signs of reinjury?
Are you afraid that you will be reinjured as soon as you return to activity?
Is there any residual swelling?
Do you feel you need a brace or other support to return to activity?

You're ready to return to activity only when you answer yes to the first three questions, and no to the latter three. (If you answered otherwise, either wait a little longer or seek the advice of a physician.)

IN CONCLUSION—A MESSAGE FOR OUR DAUGHTERS

ALTHOUGH MANY WOMEN DON'T realize it, we're all role models for the other women and girls in our lives. Each day we make choices that influence the behavior of others, especially children. Too many girls grow up constantly hearing criticisms of the female form, which makes them critical of their own developing bodies. And although the media is often blamed for our obsession with thinness, magazines and television aren't the only influences. Think about it: How often do you say something critical about your thighs, your stomach, your appearance in general? How sad that there are girls who have never heard their mothers say anything positive about this wonderful "machine" that houses us! Think what a powerful message it would send if, instead of criticizing our physical appearances, we begin teaching girls to appreciate what strong, healthy fit female bodies are capable of.

The benefits of fitness go well beyond the physical for adolescent girls. Studies show that girls who are physically active are 75 percent more likely to graduate from high school, 80 percent less likely to have unwanted pregnancies, and 90 percent less likely to be involved with drugs. It's no secret that the overwhelming majority of female CEOs say they were "tomboys" as children, and that being physically active contributed significantly to their developing self-confidence and self-esteem.

Last but not least, the health of the men and boys in your life will also benefit from your new commitment to fitness. Not only are women important role models for young girls and other women, they are also what I call the "lifestyle leaders" of the family. If you are active, your children and your spouse are likely to follow your lead. And a fit family makes for a healthier, happier one!

RESOURCES

BOOKS

The Athletic Woman's Sourcebook by Janis Graham

The Athletic Woman's Survival Guide by Carol Otis, M.D.

Eating Well for Optimum Health by Andrew Weil, M.D.

The Female Cyclist by Gale Bernhardt

How to Raise Children Without Breaking your Back by Alex Pirie and Hollis Herman, M.S., P.T.

Muscle Mechanics by Everett Aaberg

Nancy Clark's Sports Nutrition Guidebook by Nancy Clark, M.S., R.D.

The Pilates Body by Brooke Siler

Running and Walking for Women over 40 by Kathrine Switzer

Stretching by Bob and Jean Anderson

Strong Women Stay Young by Miriam E. Nelson, Ph.D.

Triathlon 101: Essentials for Multisport Success by John Mora

Weight Training for Dummies by Liz Neporent and Suzanne Schlosberg

The Whartons' Stretch Book by Jim and Phil Wharton

MAGAZINES

Cooking Light
Fitness
Health
Runner's World (has an excellent annual shoe review)
Self
Shape
Sports Illustrated Women
Weight Watchers

NEWSLETTERS

ACSM Fit Society Journal (www.acsm.org/newsletters.htm)
The Cornell Food & Fitness Advisor (800-829-2505)
The Cornell Women's Health Advisor (800-847-7131)
Georgia Tech Sports Medicine & Performance Newsletter
   (800-783-4903)
Harvard Women's Health Watch (877-388-7761 or *www.health. harvard.edu*)
Tufts University Health & Nutrition Letter (800-274-7581)

ORGANIZATIONS

American Cancer Society
PO Box 102454
Atlanta, GA 30368-2454
800-227-2345
www.cancer.org

American College of Sports Medicine
PO Box 1440
Indianapolis, IN 46206-1440
317-637-9200
www.acsm.org

American Council on Exercise
4851 Paramount Drive
San Diego, CA 92123
800-825-3636
www.acefitness.org

American Dietetic Association
216 West Jackson Blvd
Chicago, IL 60606
800-366-1655
www.eatright.org

American Heart Association
(call for regional office address)
800-242-8721
www.amhrt.org

The President's Council on Physical Fitness and Sports
HHH Building, room 738-H
200 Independence Ave S.W.
Washington, D.C. 20201-0004
202-690-9000

Women's Sports Foundation
Eisenhower Park
East Meadow, NY 11554
800-227-3988
www.womenssportsfoundation.org

ADDITIONAL WEB SITES

www.aapsm.org
The Web site of the American Academy of Podiatric Sports Medicine, which has an updated list of currently available athletic shoes designed to accommodate specific foot types.

www.active.com
A great way to find and register for a variety of events and sports participation opportunities.

www.amtamassage.org
The Web site of the American Massage Therapy Association; it has information about massage and includes a locator to help you find a licensed massage therapist in any locale.

www.drweil.com
Dr. Andrew Weil uses his extensive knowledge of alternative/integrative medicine to answer questions about health, fitness, and nutrition.

www.healthfinder.gov
Developed by the U.S. Department of Health and Human Services, this site will guide you to reliable consumer health information, including online publications, clearinghouses, databases, Web sites, and support and self-help groups.

www.nal.usda.gov/fnic
USDA Food and Nutrition Information Center

www.yogazone.com
www.yogasite.com
Good introductions to yoga; videotapes available include Pilates.

RETAIL

Athleta
High-quality athletic wear for women
888-322-5515
www.athleta.com

Collage Video
Catalog company with extensive exercise video selection; includes video-specific ratings from major fitness-oriented magazines like *Self,* *Fitness,* and *Shape*; also includes designation of "staff favorites"

800-433-6769
www.Collagevideo.com

Junonia
Great gear and advice for active women sizes 14 and up
800-586-6642
www.Junonia.com

Performance Bicycle
Its wide selection varies from bicycling apparel and shoes to heart-rate monitors and running strollers
800-727-2453
www.performancebike.com

Road Runner Sports
Running apparel, shoes, gadgets, and accessories
800-551-5558
www.roadrunnersports.com

Terry Precision Cycling
Bicycles and cycling gear designed specifically for a woman's anatomy
800-289-8379
www.terrybicycles.com

Title 9 Sports
Wide variety of athletic wear for women and girls
800-609-0092
www.titlesports.com

MISCELLANEOUS REFERENCES

"ACSM Position on the Recommended Quantity and Quality of Exercise for Developing and Maintaining Cardiorespiratory and Muscular Fitness, and Flexibility in Adults." In *Med Sci Sports Exercise,* 1998 Jun 30(6):975–91.

"Mental Health: A Report from the Surgeon General." www.surgeon general.gov/library/mentalhealth/home.html

"Physical Activity and Health: A Report of the Surgeon General." www.cdc.gov/nccdphp/sgr/summ.html

INDEX

treating, 285–93
inner thigh, exercises for, *138*
interval training, 158–60
iron, xvi, 239–41, 292

jogging, 28, 46, 49, 50
joints, 51, 82, 84, 91, 141
jump training, 191

kneecap pain, 265–67

lat pull-down, *132*
Lotte Berk method, 177
lower back, exercises for, *101–2*

magazines, 298
massage, 273
maximum heart rate (MHR), 55–58
menopause, 26, 27, 109
menstrual cycle, xvii, 216, 217, 240, 244
    cessation/interruption of, 247, 248, 249–50, 251, 265
    gender-related injuries and, 269
mental health, 43–44
minerals, in diet, 233–36
modalities, 291
money, lack of, 23–24
muscles, 107, 114, 147, 174, 224
    aging and, 106, 117
    imbalances of, 278–79
    metabolism and, 115, 208
    strain injuries to, 271–74
    variety-training and, 131
music, exercise and, 168

newsletters, 298

obesity, 41, 44, 46, 147, 218
organizations, 298–99
osteoarthritis, 46, 70, 84
osteoporosis, x, xvii, 4, 8, 25, 72
    age and, 25–26
    calcium and, 238–39
    cardiovascular exercise and, 45
    female athlete triad and, 248, 250, 251
    risk factors for, 109
    skeletal development and, 258
    strength training and, 106, 108–9, 147, 178
    weight-bearing activities and, 45, 52
outer thigh, exercises for, *136–37*
overpronation, 75
overtraining, 185–88
overuse injuries, 260–67, 275

pain, 141, 184, 256, 293
    delayed onset muscle soreness (DOMS), 148–49
    in knees, 69, 162, 179
    overtraining and, 187
    stretching and, 90, 103
"pear-shaped" pattern, 141, 219
pedometers, 48
peppermint, 238
periodization, 174–76
personal trainers, 150–51, 169
physical therapy, 290–91
Pilates method, 176–77
plyometrics, 191
pregnancy, xvii, xviii, 4, 18
    adolescent girls and, 296
    bicycling and, 162
    drugs/medications and, 289
    exercise during, xvi, 26–27

shoulders, exercises for, *94,* 127
single leg squat, 119–20, *120,* 124
smoking, 38, 46, 92, 109, 180, 211
snacks, 232–33
sports, 188–98
sports bras, 197
sprains, 268–69
stair steppers, 164, 209
steroids, 236
strains, 270–74
strength training (weight lifting), xvi, xx, 11, 25, 105–6,
    122–24
  aging and, 116–18
  alternate methods of, 176–77
  avoiding injuries and, 280
  bone health and, 108–9
  breaking barriers to, 111–12
  burning calories and, 207
  designing programs for, 118–21, 141–43
  diet and, 152
  expectations from, 147–48
  fitness factors and, 125–31
  health benefits of, 110–11
  medical conditions and, 29
  muscle soreness and, 148–49
  muscle strength vs. endurance, 121–22
  myths and realities about, 112–14
  periodization and, 174–76
  personal trainers and, 150–51
  pregnancy and, 27
  sample exercises, *132–40*
  sample programs, 143–47
stress fractures, 263–65
stress relief, 7, 18, 45, 103
stretching, 28, 69, 82, 276–77, 280–81